Comprehensive Review of Oral Medicine

Comprehensive Review of Oral Medicine

Pramod John R.
B.Sc., B.D.S., M.D.S.
Professor & Head of Department,
Department of Oral Medicine and Radiology,
Amrita College of Dentistry,
Amrita Institute of Medical Sciences & Research Centre,
Cochin - 682 026, Kerala (India)

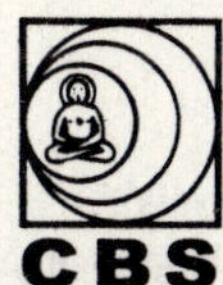

CBS PUBLISHERS & DISTRIBUTORS
NEW DELHI • BANGALORE

ISBN : 81-239-1224-2

First Edition : 2005

Publishing Director : Vinod K. Jain

Published by :
Satish Kumar Jain for CBS Publishers & Distributors,
4596/1-A, 11 Darya Ganj, New Delhi - 110 002 (India)
E-mail : cbspubs@del3.vsnl.net.in
Website : http://www.cbspd.com

Branch Office :
2975, 17th Cross, K.R. Road,
Bansankari 2nd Stage, Bangalore - 560070
Fax : 080-26771680 • E-mail : cbsbng@vsnl.net

Printed at :
Asia Printograph, Delhi

PREFACE

This book, titled, 'Comprehensive Review of Oral Medicine' has been written as a study material for those who are preparing for the postgraduate entrance examinations of various Indian Universities. Now majority of the universities have adopted entrance examination with multiple choice questions as the mode of examination. As the time available in the exhaustive preparation for the entrance examination is minimal and there is a requirement to go through enormous amount of study material, a comprehensive review of the subject concerned would greatly benefit the reader in his/her preparation in the short and available time.

This book has been intended for use by the graduate dental student who is aspiring for a postgraduate course. The book includes multiple choice questions and brief notes wherever required so that the reader would get adequate information about the subject in the limited time available. It is my strong belief that I have tried to cover the entire length and breadth of the vast subject of Oral Medicine. My many years of teaching experience as well as expertise in having prepared multiple choice questions for postgraduate entrance examinations of various Indian Universities have been used in the preparation of this book. I am sure that this book would greatly help the readers who are aiming for new horizons of learning.

I request the readers to kindly offer criticisms, suggestions or opinions about the book. I wish all the readers the very best in their efforts in pursuing a postgraduate degree.

Pramod John

CONTENTS

Preface v

How to Prepare for P.G. Entrance Examination and How to Answer the Multiple Choice Questions ix

Section I 1
Section II 17
Section III 33
Section IV 48
Section V 65
Section VI 84
Section VII 100
Section VIII 116
Section IX 131
Section X 147
Section XI 161

HOW TO PREPARE FOR P.G. ENTRANCE EXAMINATION AND HOW TO ANSWER THE MULTIPLE CHOICE QUESTIONS

Practically all the postgraduate institutions are now conducting entrance examinations for admitting candidates for postgraduate courses and multiple choice questions are the main mode by which these tests are conducted. This is an effective way of assessing the candidates without any bias or examiner variability factor. Yet another advantage is MCQs generally help in assessing the recall knowledge of the students. It must also be emphasized that valuation of the answer papers is also easier because if the key to the answers is given, even a person without any knowledge of the subject can value the answer papers.

The crucial step in facing the challenge of the P.G. entrance examination lies in preparing for the examination well in advance. It has been widely assumed that sheer luck and statistical probability factors greatly influenze the success in the examination. This is based on the fact that if an MCQ questionnaire is given to a person who has not studied the subject he can still randomly choose answers and statistically still he would be capable of scoring marks, even 100% marks! Having said that, it must be stressed that a candidate preparing for P.G. entrance examination must not rely too much on the luck factor and must put in a genuine effort to prepare for it.

Three to six months of intense preparation is imperative to face the entrance examination. It goes without saying that a thorough grasp of the subjects is essential to write the test well.

The following steps may be useful for the preparation and writing of P.G. entrance examination:

- Start your preparation at least six months in advance.
- Allocate sufficient time for study every day.
- Plan your studies properly.
- Set a target for covering the study material (for example you should be able to cover at least four chapters of the text every day).
- After reading the standard textbooks available, try to work out the multiple choice questions. Perhaps it would be wise to cover the MCQs subjectwise.
- Go through each question carefully and try to answer on your own.
- In case you are unable to recollect the answer, refer the key.

- You can use separate sheets for writing your answers and in the end, compare your answers with the key.
- Repeat the tests periodically and evaluate your score.
- When you face the real entrance examination, go with a relaxed mind.
- Answer each question as fast as you could and never waste your time in each question.
- If you have sufficient time, come back to the question and try to answer.
- As most of the P.G. entrance examinations penalize for wrong answers, if you are not sure of the answer, never attempt it.
- Intelligent guess in answering a question not familiar with is desirable, but at the same time make sure that it is not a wild guess which would take away your score.

SECTION I

1. What is diagnosis?

   Diagnosis refers to the process by which the patient's health as well as the opinions formulated by the clinician after taking the case history and clinical examination are evaluated.

2. What is Oral Diagnosis?

   Oral Diagnosis refers to the art of using scientific knowledge to diagnose disease processes affecting the oral and related structures and to distinguish one disease from the other.

3. What is Oral Medicine?

   Oral Medicine is that area of dental science that deals with diagnosis and treatment of diseases affecting the oral cavity which may either be present locally or which are oral manifestations of systemic diseases and it also deals with those phases of dentistry which is essentially concerned with the management of medically compromised patients who present with dental problems.

4. What are oral diseases?

   Oral diseases refer to those diseases which are either localized in the oral cavity or which are oral manifestations of systemic diseases.

5. What are the principles of examination?

   Principles of examination refers to the methods by which clinical examination is conducted.

   Inspection: Inspection refers to systematic visual appraisal of the patient during physical examination. This is the preliminary step in the process of physical examination. By performing a thorough inspection any obvious signs of the disease will be discernible to the clinician.

   Palpation: Palpation refers to the method of examination of structures or parts of the body or any pathology by feeling or pressing. Palpation helps in finding out the following changes:

   - Temperature changes
   - Tenderness
   - Consistency of the pathology

- Assessment of fixity or movability of the pathology
- Assessment of the periphery of the pathology
- Assessment of fractures

Percussion: Percussion refers to the method of using instruments or fingers to assess the sound that is generated when struck on structures. Percussion has an important role to play in assessing tenderness of teeth.

Auscultation: Auscultation refers to the use of a stethoscope in order to enhance the sound arising from the heart, lungs as well as from the temporomandibular joint.

Diascopy: One of the features of vascular (blood-containing) lesions is that when pressure is applied to the lesion, blanching occurs. The method of using a glass slide to compress the lesion is known as diascopy. The blanching occurs because of forceful removal of blood from these lesions when pressure is applied.

Probing: Probing refers to the use of a slender instrument called probe or explorer in order to assess the extent of a tract or cavity. Probing has special role to play in the detection of caries as well as in the assessment of periodontal pocket depth.

6. Bradycardia can be caused by all except:
   a. Myxoedema
   b. Jaundice
   c. Raised intracranial pressure
   d. Thyrotoxicosis
7. Blood pressure is elevated in all the conditions except:
   a. Cushing's syndrome
   b. Phaeochromocytoma
   c. Coarctation of aorta
   d. Shock
8. Normal oral temperature is:
   a. 37°C
   b. 37°F
   c. 27°C
   d. 27°F
9. Respiratory rate is increased by all except:
   a. Narcotic drug therapy
   b. Exercise
   c. Fever
   d. Thyrotoxicosis
10. Diascopy is performed in case of
    a. Vascular lesions
    b. Bony hard lesions
    c. Lymph node examination
    d. Salivary gland studies

Ans. 6. d 7. d 8. a 9. a 10. a

11. Purpura contains
    a. Melanine pigmentation
    b. Blood
    c. Endogenous pigmented substances
    d. Iron

12. Petechiae are examples for
    a. Vesicle
    b. Bulla
    c. Macule
    d. Papule

13. Pathological calcification occurring in degenerating and dead tissues is called
    a. Dystrophic calcification
    b. Calcinosis
    c. Hypercalcemia
    d. Hypertrophic ossification

14. Most oral bacteria grow best when the pH is
    a. 7
    b. Acidic
    c. Alkaline
    d. Unaffected by pH

15. Epstein-Barr virus causes
    a. Common cold
    b. Epstein pearls
    c. Lupus erythematosus
    d. Infectious mononucleosis

16. Sialorrhea can occur as a result of all except
    a. Oral cancer
    b. Familial autonomic dysfunction
    c. Sarcoidosis
    d. Teething

17. State true or false: Statistically boys are affected more often by clefts.
    a. T
    b. F

18. What are the causes for macroglossia or enlarged tongue?
    - Overdevelopment of the tongue musculature
    - Beckwith's hypoglycemic syndrome
    - Amyloidosis
    - Hurler's syndrome

Ans. 11. b 12. c 13. a 14. a 15. d 16. c 17. T

- Cretinism
- Hyperpituitarism
- Hemangioma
- Lymphangioma
- Neurofibroma
- Obstruction of lymphatic drainage in case of malignancy

19. What are the causes for angular cheilitis (cheilosis or perleché)
    - Atropic dermatitis
    - Increased fold formation as a result of ageing
    - Overclosure among complete denture-wearers due to decreased vertical dimension
    - Pooling of saliva in the corners of the mouth due to increased salivation
    - Nutritional deficiencies
    - Xerostomia
    - Starvation
    - Anemia
    - Acute and chronic systemic diseases
    - Allergic conditions
    - Mechanical overstretching of the mouth as during dental procedures

20. Among the following, which is not a feature of Pierre Robin syndrome?
    a. Glossoptosis b. Micrognathia
    c. Cleft palate d. Glossodynia

21. Leontiasis ossea can cause
    a. micrognathia b. Macrognathia
    c. Cleft palate d. Facial edema

22. Apert's syndrome is characterized by all except:
    a. Craniostenosis b. Exophthalmos
    c. Syndactyly d. Fissured tongue

23. Treacher-Collin's syndrome is characterized by all except:
    a. Craniostenosis b. Malformed ear
    c. Ocular abnormalities d. Large mouth

24. Cleavage of a tooth germ during early development results in
    a. Fusion b. Gemination
    c. Dilaceration d. Taurodontism

Ans. 20. d 21. b 22. d 23. a 24. b

25. Enamel hypoplasia can occur as a result of all except:
   a. Paget's disease
   b. Rh hemolytic disease
   c. German measles
   d. Congenital syphilis

26. "Ghost teeth" refer to which condition
   a. Treacher-Collin syndrome
   b. Regional odontodysplasia
   c. Amelogenesis imperfecta
   d. Dentinogenesis imperfecta

27. Diffuse swellings occurring in the lips is a feature of
   a. Wegener's granulomatosis
   b. Meisher's syndrome
   c. Treacher-Collin syndrome
   d. Apert syndrome

28. Fordyce granules refer to
   a. Sebaceous glands
   b. Sweat glands
   c. Hair follicles
   d. Fat cells

29. "Butterfly-like" configuration of angiofibroma is seen in all the following except:
   a. Tuberous sclerosis
   b. Discoid lupus erythematosus
   c. Familial dysautonomia

30. The consistency of lymph nodes in lymphoma is described as
   a. Soft
   b. Rubbery
   c. Stony hard
   d. Firm

31. Chemical substances responsible for halitosis are:
   a. Hydrogen sulphide and methyl mercaptan
   b. Hydrogen peroxide and methyl carbide
   c. Carbon monoxide and hydrocarbons
   d. Nitrous oxide and sulphur

32. Mucocutaneos lymph node syndrome is considered to be caused by:
   a. Bacteria
   b. Fungi
   c. Rickettsiae
   d. Virus

33. The main causative organism of dental caries is
   a. Streptococcus mutans
   b. Streptococcus viridans
   c. Actinomyces
   d. Staphylococcus aureus

Ans. 25. a 26. b 27. b 28. a 29. c 30. b 31. a 32. c
33. a

34. Microscopically, presence of parakeratosis and extensive spongiosis are features of
    a. Cheilitis glandularis
    b. White sponge nevus
    c. Macrocheilia
    d. Macrostomia
35. Nursing bottle caries mainly affects
    a. Maxillary central incisors
    b. Mandibular incisors
    c. Maxillary molars
    d. Mandibular molars
36. An arrested caries is diagnosed by
    a. Absence of softness
    b. Blackish discolouration
    c. Chalky white area
    d. "Catch" on probing
37. Removal of pulp tissue results in the loss of translucency of the teeth because of
    a. Dehydration of the tooth
    b. Loss of enamel
    c. Resorption of dentin
    d. Inability of light to penetrate the hard tissue structure
38. Among the following drugs, which drug is not associated with causing gingival enlargement
    a. Cyclosporine
    b. Nifedipine
    c. Phenytoin sodium
    d. Oxyphenbutazone
39. Among smokers gingival inflammation can occur because
    a. Tobacco is an irritant to the gingiva
    b. Physical injury caused by cigarette
    c. Nicotine from tobacco is an irritant
    d. Frequent drying and moistening of the gingiva
40. Among the following statements about diffuse gingival fibromatosis, which is correct?
    a. Familial occurrence
    b. Caused by drugs
    c. Inflammation is the main etological factor
    d. Predominantly seen among mouth breathers

Ans. 34. b 35. a 36. a 37. a 38. d 39. d 40. a

41. Among the following syndromes which is not associated with gingival enlargement
    a. Cowden's syndrome
    b. Cross syndrome
    c. Reiter's syndrome
    d. Rutherford syndrome

42. Bohn's nodules are seen in
    a. Newborn
    b. Complete denture wearers
    c. Oral cancer patients
    d. Pregnant women

43. The usual location of Epstein's pearl is
    a. Lower lip
    b. Along the midpalatine raphae
    c. Tongue
    d. Buccal mucosa and gingiva

44. Epstein's pearl is a
    a. Bony enlargement
    b. Fibrotic overgrowth
    c. Inflammatory edema
    d. Keratin-filled cyst

45. The etiology of Wegener's granulomatosis is
    a. Unknown causes
    b. Due to bacteria
    c. Immunosuppressive therapy
    d. Heredity

46. Pain on lying down in acute pulpitis is due to
    a. Increased temperature
    b. Decreased metabolic activity during sleep
    c. Compression by the tongue
    d. Congestion of apical vasculature

47. Lateral periodontal cyst occurs in the
    a. Molar region　　b. Premolar region
    c. Incisor region　　d. Canine region

Ans. 41. c 42. a 43. b 44. b 45. a 46. d 47. b

48. Acute necrotizing ulcerative gingivostomatitis (ANUG) is caused by
    a. Bacteroides fragilis
    b. Borrelia vincentii
    c. Endobacter
    d. Streptococcus viridans

49. Ectodermal dysplasia is characterized by
    a. Hypohidrosis, hypotrichosis and hypodontia
    b. Hypotelorism, hypodontia and hypotension
    c. Hypohidrosis, hypoplasia and hypotelorism
    d. Hypodontia, hypovascularity and hypopituitarism

50. Fissured tongue is a feature of
    a. Peutz Jeghers syndrome
    b. Darier-White disease
    c. Melkersson Rosenthal syndrome
    d. Albright's syndrome

51. Unusual extensibility of the tongue is called
    a. Lingual varicosity
    b. Elastic tongue
    c. Rubbery tongue
    d. Gorlin sign

52. Which are the drugs associated with gingival enlargement?

    The common drugs associated with gingival enlargement as a side-effect are the following:

    - Phenytoin sodium (dilantin sodium) which is an antiepileptic drug and also sometimes used in the treatment of trigeminal neuralgia in conjunction with baclofen
    - Nifedipine which is a calcium channel blocker used in the treatment of hypertension
    - Cyclosporine which is a potent immunosuppressive drug which is used after organ transplantation
    - Antianxiety drugs such as barbiturates
    - Prolonged use of oral contraceptive drugs

53. The cyst which occurs due to the cystic degeneration and liquefaction of stellate reticulum in an enamel organ before calcification is called
    a. Lateral periodontal cyst
    b. Primordial cyst
    c. Perapical cyst
    d. Globulomaxillary cyst

Ans. 48. b 49. a 50. c 51. d 53. b

54. Large blood-filled spaces lined by spindle-shaped cells is a feature of
 a. Radicular cyst
 b. Residual cyst
 c. Aneurysmal bone cyst
 d. Globulomaxillary cyst

55. Lupus vulgaris refers to:
 a. Lesion associated with systemic lupus erythematosus
 b. Tuberculous infection involving the skin
 c. Syphilitic lesion involving the skin
 d. Skin involvement in AIDS

56. A cyst is defined as a pathological cavity, lined by epithelium and containing solid, semisolid, or gaseous substance but not pus. Cysts are classified as given below:
 1. True cysts
  A. Odontogenic
   a. Inflammatory
    Periapical
   b. Developmental
    i. Primordial
    ii. Gingival
    iii. Eruption
    iv. Lateral periodontal
    v. Dentigerous.
  B. Non-odontogenic
   i. Incisive canal
   ii. Median palatine
   iii. Nasolabial
   iv. Globulomaxillary
 2. False cysts
  i. Traumatic bone
  ii. Aneurysmal bone

 Frequency of occurrence of various cyst types is given below:

1. Radicular (periapical)	: 65%
2. Dentigerous	: 15%
3. Nasopalatine	: 8%
4. Primordial	: 7%
5. Solitary bone	: 2%

Ans. 54. c 55. b

6. Nasolabial : 0.5%
7. Lateral periodontal : 0.3%
8. Gingival cyst : 0.1%
9. Aneurysmal bone : 0.1%

57. Which stage of syphilis is associated with mucous patches
    a. Primary
    b. Secondary
    c. Tertiary
    d. Latent

58. Diagnosis of tuberculosis is made by
    a. Reiter's test
    b. Kveim-Siltzbach test
    c. Mantoux test
    d. L.E. test

59. Jarrisch-Herxheimer reaction can occur following treatment of
    a. Syphilis
    b. Leprosy
    c. Tuberculosis
    d. Cervicofacial actinomycosis

60. Presence of "sulphur granules" in the pus is a feature of
    a. Syphilis
    b. Leprosy
    c. Tuberculosis
    d. Cervicofacial actinomycosis

61. "Ray fungus" is a term given for
    a. Candida albicans
    b. Actinomyces israelii
    c. Borrelia vincentii
    d. Treponema pallidum

62. "Strawberry tongue" is a manifestation of
    a. Diphtheria
    b. Gonococcal stomatitis
    c. Scarlet fever
    d. Hansen's disease

63. "Risus sardoniccus" appearance is a feature of
    a. Diphthera
    b. Scarlet fever
    c. Tetanus
    d. Gonococcal stomatitis

Ans. 57. b 58. c 59. a 60. d 61. b 62. c 63. c

64. A complication of acute necrotizing ulcerative gingivostomatitis is

a. Osteomyelitis
b. Actinomycosis
c. Cancrum oris
d. Gingival abscess

65. Detection of sequestrum on radiographic examination is a feature of

a. Osteogenic sarcoma
b. Hyperparathyroidism
c. Tori
d. Osteomyelitis

66. Condensing osteitis is also called as

a. Diffuse sclerosing osteomyelitis
b. Focal sclerosing osteomyelitis
c. Suppurative osteomyelitis
d. Garré's osteomyelitis

67. "Onion peel" appearance on radiographic examination is a feature of

a. Garré's osteomyelitis
b. Multiple myeloma
c. Sickle cell anemia
d. Paget's disease

68. Notes : The lesions associated with "onion peel" appearance on radiographic examination are the following:

- Tori
- Exostoses
- Peripheral osteoma
- Ewing's sarcoma
- Infantile cortical hyperostosis
- Fibrous dysplasia
- Osteosarcoma
- Ossifying subperosteal hematoma
- Callus formation after fracture

69. The virus associated with the etiology of nasopharyngeal carcinoma is

a. Epstein-Barr
b. Herpes simplex
c. Varicella zoster
d. Cytomegalovirus

Ans. 64. c 65. d 66. b 67. a 69. d

70. A diagnostic test for the diagnosis of herpetic gingivostomatitis is
    a. Viral culture
    b. Tzanck smear
    c. Mono spot test
    d. Compliment fixation test

71. Diseases associated with aphthous ulcers are the following except:
    a. Behçet's disease
    b. Crohn's disease
    c. Gluten-sensitive enteropathy
    d. Eosinophilic granuloma

72. Notes : Recurrent aphthous ulcers (RAU) are also called as recurrent aphthous stomatitis or "canker sore". These are painful ulcers which occur in the non-keratinized oral epithelium and usually require 8-14 days for healing depending on the size and location of the lesion. The exact etiological factors associated with RAU are not known. However, the role of the following factors have been proposed. These factors are:

- Stress
- Allegic
- Microbial
- Traumatic
- Nutritional deficiencies (mainly deficiency of iron vitamin B complex etc.)
- Endocrine
- Hereditary
- Autoimmune

Usually RAU affects individuals in the second decade. Clinically RAU is divided into the following types:

RAU minor: RAU minor lesions are usually 2-3 mm in size

RAU major: RAU major lesions are more than 3 mm in size. These lesions can persist even up to 6 weeks.

Recurrent herpetiform ulcerations: RAU lesions of the herpetiform type appear as clusters and clinically may mimic herpetic lesions.

RAU associated with Behcet's syndrome: This syndrome is characterized by involvement of oral mucosa, eyes as well as genitals.

Ans. 70. b 71. d

73. Deep fissures are called

a. Urticaria
b. Rhagades
c. Atrophy
d. Papule

74. A flat spot less than 1 cm in diameter is called

a. Macule
b. Papule
c. Patch
d. Pustule

75. The following statements about *epulis gravidarum* are correct except

a. Occurs in pregnant women
b. It is a tumor-like granulomatous lesion
c. It is a reactive proliferation of blood vessels
d. It is a feature of eosinophilic granuloma

76. Pebbly appearance of the lower lip is termed

a. Cheilitis glandularis
b. Angular cheilitis
c. Macrocheilia
d. Exfoliative cheilitis

77. Black hairy tongue occurs due to

a. Ectopic growth of hair on the tongue
b. Hyperkeratotic papillae
c. Skin grafting on the tongue
d. Excessive stimulation of hair growth

78. Pyostomatitis vegetans has a strong association with

a. Rhematoid arthritis
b. Ulcerative colitis
c. Behçet's syndrome
d. Stevens-Johnson syndrome

79. Pigmentation associated with pregnancy is called

a. Chloasma
b. Chloroma
c. Chlorophylia
d. Cheilosis

80. An endocrine disorder associated with pigmentation is

a. Hyperadrenocorticism
b. Addison's disease
c. Diabetes mellitus
d. Cushing's syndrome

81. Among the following which is not associated with endogenous pigmentation

a. Whipple's syndrome
b. Peutz-Jegher's syndrome
c. Hemochromatosis
d. Heck's disease

Ans. 73. b 74. a 75. d 76. a 77. b 78. b 79. a 80. b
81. d

82. The drug associated with pigmentation is
    a. Antimalarials
    b. Antihypertensives
    c. Oral hypoglycemic drugs
    d. Immunosuppressive drugs

83. Lack of the enzyme C1-INH can cause
    a. Hereditary angioedema
    b. White sponge nevus
    c. Lupus erythematosus
    d. Growth retardation

84. Koebner's phenomenon is a feature of
    a. Lichen planus
    b. Recurrent aphthous stomatitis
    c. Psoriasis
    d. Erythema multiforme

85. Benign migratory glossitis is considered to be a variant of
    a. Psoriasis
    b. Lichen planus
    c. Erythema multiforme
    d. Pemphigus

86. ——— is not a feature of Reiter's disease
    a. Arthritis
    b. Urethritis
    c. Conjunctivitis
    d. Dermatitis

87. Reiter's syndrome may be treated with all the following except:
    a. Corticosteroids
    b. NSAIDs
    c. Methotrexate
    d. Retinoids

88. Among the following ——— is not a feature of rosacea
    a. Telangiectases
    b. Sebaceous gland hyperplasia
    c. Perivascular fibrosis
    d. Conjunctivitis

Ans. 82. a 83. a 84. c 85. a 86. d 87. a 88. d

89. ——— is not a feature of Sweet's syndrome

a. High incidence of dental caries
b. Fever
c. Malaise
d. Erythematous nodules

90. Benign mucous membranous pemphigoid is also called as

a. Bullous pemphigoid
b. Cicatricial pemphigoid
c. Pemphigus vegetans
d. Pemphigus foliaceous

91. Black hairy tongue

- Cause is unknown
- Microbial etiology (probably)
- Imbalance in the oral microbial flora
- Predisposed by the use of drugs such as the following
  - Penicillin
  - Cephalosporin
  - Tetracyclin
  - Chloramphenicol
  - Streptomycin
  - Isoniazid
  - Metronidazole
  - Griseofulvin

92. Herpangina is caused by

a. Coxsackievirus
b. Herpes simplex virus
c. Cytomegalovirus
d. Paramyxovirus

93. Among the following statements about herpangina which one is incorrect?

a. It is a disease of the childhood
b. It occurs as epidemics
c. Lesions appear as multiple blisters
d. Affects mainly anterior part of the mouth

94. Photophobia is a feature of

a. Herpes zoster
b. Measles
c. Mumps
d. Infectious mononucleosis

Ans. 89. a 90. b 92. a 93. d 94. b

95. Presence of Koplik's spots is a characteristic feature of
    a. Rubella
    b. Mumps
    c. Infectious mononucleosis
    d. Measles

96. Subepithelial bulla formation is a feature of
    a. Lichen planus
    b. Oral submucous fibrosis
    c. Cicatricial pemphigoid
    d. Leukoplakia

97. Necrotizing sialometaplasia is thought to be caused by
    a. A compromise in the blood supply to the salivary glands
    b. Viral infection
    c. Bacterial infection
    d. Malignant transformation of salivary gland

98. Spontaneous oral bleeding can occur if the platelet count falls below —— mm^3
    a. 50,000
    b. 1,00,000
    c. 2,00,000
    d. Unaffected by fall in the platelet count

99. Thrombocytopenia may be associated with all except:
    a. Sjögren's syndrome
    b. Systemic lupus erythematosus
    c. Felty's syndrome
    d. Pemphigus foliaceous

100. Children usually do not get herpetic gingivostomatitis before the age of 6 months because:
    a. Virus cannot survive in infant's mouth
    b. Maternal antibodies provide resistance
    c. Oral cavity is sterile in infants
    d. Oral bacteria suppress the growth of viruses

Ans. 95. d 96. c 97. a 98. a 99. d 100. b

SECTION II

1. Oral candidiasis is classified as given below.

   Acute
   Acute pseudomemranous candidiasis
   Acute atrophic candidiasis
   Angular cheilitis
   Chronic
   Chronic atrophic candidiasis
   Chronic hyperplastic candidiasis
   Mucocutaneous candidiasis
   Localized type
   Familial type
   Syndromes associated with candidiasis

2. What are the etiological factors for candidiasis?

   Oral candidiasis is a fungal infection caused by the fungus, *Candida albicans*. It is a normal commensal in the oral cavity even in normal individuals. In smaller numbers it does not cause any disease. Its growth and multiplication are also suppressed by other oral bacteria. However, its count increases when the resistance of the host falls due to a variety of factors.

   - Physiological factors such as age (in children as well as the elderly)
   - Genetic predisposition
   - Hormonal factors such as hypoparathyroidism, diabetes mellitus and Addison's disease
   - Iatrogenic facors such as prolonged use of broad-spectrum antibiotics, chemotherapy for the treatment of malignancy, radiotherapy and immunosuppressive therapy
   - Systemic factors such as carcinoma, rheumatoid arthritis, lupus erythematosus, iron deficiency, pernicious anemia, lichen planus, AIDS and certain hereditary disorders associated with altered immune response
   - Local factors such as use of dentures, angular cheilitis, overclosure of the mouth, leukoplakia etc.

3. Incidence of tori is high among which race?
   a. Negroid
   b. Eskimos
   c. Chinese
   d. Caucasians
4. What are the causes for hemifacial hypertrophy?
   - The exact etiology is not known
   - Incomplete twinning
   - Hormonal imbalance
   - Alterations in the intrauterine development
   - Vascular or lymphatic abnormalities
5. Fusion of two independently formed teeth with cementum is called:
   a. Taurodontism
   b. Concrescence
   c. Fusion
   d. Gemination
6. A syndrome associated with multiple unerupted supernumerary teeth is:
   a. Sjögren's syndrome
   b. Gardner's syndrome
   c. Rutherford's syndrome
   d. Klinefelter's syndrome
7. Presence of "sulphur granules" in the pus is suggestive of:
   a. Actinomycosis
   b. Osteomyelitis
   c. Osteoradionecrosis
   d. Metastatic jaw lesion
8. Jarisch-Herxheimer reaction refers to:
   a. Reaction to penicillin
   b. Reaction to sulphonamides
   c. Exacerbation of local syphilitic lesion following treatment
   d. Vascular eruptions following cancer treatment
9. Mucous patches are characteristic of which stage of syphilis?
   a. Primary
   b. Secondary
   c. Tertiary
   d. Congenital
10. Chancre is a syphilitic lesion occurring in which stage of syphilis?
    a. Primary
    b. Secondary
    c. Tertiary
    d. Congenital

Ans. 3. c 5. b 6. b 7. d 8. c 9. b 10. a

11. What is Hutchinson's triad?
Stigmata of syphilis is characterized by involvement of bone and teeth. Hutchinson's triad refers to the following features:
- Hypoplasia of incisors and first permanent molars
- VIII nerve deafness
- Interstitial keratitis

12. "Leutic tongue" is a feature of:
a. Tertiary syphilis
b. Tuberculosis
c. Leprosy
d. Leukoplakia

13. "Split papules" occur in:
a. Tuberculosis
b. Leprosy
c. Verrucous carcinoma
d. Secondary syphilis

14. Which are the clinical types of leprosy?
- Tuberculoid leprosy
- Lepromatous leprosy
- Borderline tuberculoid leprosy
- Borderline or dimorphous leprosy
- Borderline lepromatous leprosy

15. "Strawberry tongue" is a feature of:
a. Leprosy
b. Tuberculosis
c. Scarlet fever
d. Tongue cancer

16. "Wash-leather" elevated membrane of the tonsil is a feature of:
a. Leprosy
b. Tuberculosis
c. Diphtheria
d. Scarlet fever

17. "Risus sardonicus" is a feature of:
a. Tetanus
b. Scleroderma
c. Congenital syphilis
d. Myositis ossificans

18. Noma is considered to be a complication of:
a. ANUG
b. Aphthous ulcers
c. Trigeminal neuralgia
d. HSV infection

19. What is osteomyelitis?
Osteomyelitis is an inflammatory disease of the bone which begins as an infection of the medullary cavity and haversian system and then extends to involve the periosteum of the affected bone.

Ans. 12. a 13. d 15. c 16. c 17. a 18. a

Causes :

- Lowered host resistance
- High virulence of the organism
- Malnourishment
- Diabetes mellitus
- Sickle cell disease
- Blood dyscrasias
- Myeloproliferative disorders
- Radiotherapy
- Decreased jaw vascularity
- Tuberculosis
- Osteopetrosis
- Paget's disease

20. "Onion skin" appearance is seen in all the following except:
    a. Ewing's sarcoma
    b. Caffey's disease
    c. Albright's syndrome
    d. Ossifying subperiosteal hematoma

21. A diagnostic test which can be used for the diagnosis of herpetic lesions is:
    a. Antinuclear antibody test
    b. Tzanck test
    c. Kveim-Siltzbach test
    d. Kahn test

22. A diagnostic test for Sarcoidosis is:
    a. Antinuclear antibody test
    b. Tzanck test
    c. Kveim-Siltzbach test
    d. Kahn test

23. Presence of multinucleated giant cells and ballooning degeneration on microscopic examination are suggestive of:
    a. Herpetic lesions
    b. Multiple myeloma
    c. Tuberculosis
    d. Syphilis

Ans. 20. c 21. b 22. c 23. a

24. Among the following statements about herpangina which is correct?
   a. Occurs in pregnant women
   b. Occurs in the elderly
   c. Occurs in children under 4 years of age
   d. Occurs in immunosuppressed individuals

25. Mono spot test is used in the diagnosis of:
   a. Infectious mononucleosis
   b. Syphilis
   c. Pneumonia
   d. Tuberculosis

26. 'Thrush' is also called as:
   a. Acute atrophic candidiasis
   b. Acute pseudomembranous candidiasis
   c. Chronic atrophic candidiasis
   d. Chronic hyperplastic candidiasis

27. Serum agglutination titre may be used in the diagnosis of:
   a. Systemic candidiasis
   b. Thrombocytopenic purpura
   c. Rheumatoid arthritis
   d. Rh incompatibility

28. Antibiotic sore mouth refers to:
   a. Acute pseudomembranous candidiasis
   b. Acute atrophic candidiasis
   c. Chronic atrophic candidiasis
   d. Chronic hyperplastic candidiasis

29. "Id reaction" is seen in:
   a. Candidiasis
   b. ITP
   c. Syphilis
   d. Allergy to sulphonamides

30. Preicteric phase of hepatitis B refers to:
   a. Prodromal phase
   b. Recovery phase
   c. Infectious stage
   d. Cured phase

Ans. 24. c 25. a 26. b 27. a 28. b 29. a 30. a

31. Normal plasma bilirubin level is:
    a. 0.3 mg/dl
    b. 3 .0 mg/dl
    c. 30.0 mg/dl
    d. 300.0 mg/dl

32. Complete recovery after hepatitis B occurs within:
    a. 4 days
    b. 4 weeks
    c. 4 months
    d. 4 years

33. Prothrombin (PT) above 20 seconds is suggestive of:
    a. Severe liver disease
    b. Hemophilia
    c. Platelet dysfunction
    d. Idiopathic thrombocytopenic purpura (ITP)

34. Presence of Australia Antigen in the serum is suggestive of:
    a. Hepatitis B
    b. Leukoplakia
    c. Lichen planus
    d. AIDS

35. Incubation period of hepatitis B is
    a. 2-6 days
    b. 2-6 weeks
    c. 2-6 months
    d. 2-6 years

36. Delta hepatitis is considered to be:
    a. Complication of hepatitis B
    b. Complication of hepatitis A
    c. Initial infection of hepatitis B
    d. Initial infection of hepatitis A

37. Corticosteroids are potent
    a. Antiinflammatory agents
    b. Antiparasitic agents
    c. Anticonvulsants
    d. Antipyretic agents

38. Among the following, which is not an action of corticosteroids?
    a. Alteration of vascular response to injury
    b. Decreasing capillary dilatation and permeability
    c. Prevention of release of kinins
    d. Suppression of adenylcyclase by catecholamines

39. Among the following, — is not a contraindication for corticosteroids:
    a. Tuberculosis
    b. Diabetes mellitus
    c. Hypertension
    d. Ulcerative colitis

Ans. 31. b 32. b 33. a 34. a 35. b 36. a 37. a 38. d 39. d

40. Among the following, which is not a metabolic reaction not associated with corticosteroid therapy?

a. Decreasing gluconeogenesis
b. Opposing the action of insulin
c. Increasing sodium retention
d. Increasing excretion of potassium

41. A cytologic change that can occur in association with corticosteroid therapy is:

a. Eosinophilia
b. Thrombocytopenia
c. Megaloblastic anemia
d. Anisocytosis

42. Among the following adverse effects, which is not associated with long-term therapy with corticosteroids?

a. Weight loss
b. Deposition of fat
c. Osteoporosis
d. Edema

43. What are the indications of corticosteroids?

- Aphthous ulcerations
- Lichen planus
- Pemphigus
- Oral submucous fibrosis
- Erythema multiforme
- Sinusitis

44. What are the contraindications of corticosteroid therapy?

- Tuberculosis
- Pregnancy
- Local or systemic infections
- Diabetes mellitus
- Active peptic ulcer
- Renal dysfunction
- Hypertension
- Severe cardiac diseases with decompensation such as congestive heart failure
- Glaucoma
- Myasthenia gravis
- Thromboembolic disorders
- Osteoporosis

Ans. 40. a 41. d 42. a

45. Long-term sun exposure is likely to cause:
    a. Actinic keratosis
    b. Herpes zoster
    c. Lichen planus
    d. Actinomycosis
46. Actinic keratosis usually occurs on the
    a. Buccal mucosa
    b. Palatal mucosa
    c. Corners of the mouth
    d. Vermilion border of the lower lip
47. Among the following which drug is used in the treatment of actinic keratosis?
    a. Methotrexate
    b. 5-fluorouracil
    c. Bleomycin
    d. Adriamycin
48. Nicotine stomatitis usually occurs on:
    a. Lips
    b. Tongue
    c. Palate
    d. Buccal mucosa
49. The reason suggested for the etiology of nicotine stomatitis is:
    a. Concentrated amount of hot smoke
    b. Chemical changes induced by tobacco
    c. Physical trauma
    d. Opportunistic infection such as candidiasis
50. Slightly elevated papule with punctate red centers in stomatitis nicotina palati are:
    a. Metastatically altered minor salivary gland ducts
    b. Metastatically altered sebaceous glands
    c. Inflamed capillary ducts
    d. Metastatically altered epithelial cells
51. Among the following statements about the histopathological features of stomatitis nicotina palati which is incorrect?
    a. Surface epithelium exhibits hyperkeratosis
    b. Metaplasia and hyperplasia of the minor salivary gland ducts
    c. Scattered chronic inflammation subjacent to minor salivary glands and connective tissue
    d. Atypical and dysplastic changes
52. One of the side-effects of using sanguinaria-containing mouthwash is:
    a. Oral candidiasis
    b. Leukoplakia-like lesions
    c. Allergic stomatitis
    d. Burns

Ans. 45. a 46. d 47. b 48. c 49. a 50. a 51. d 52. b

53. Oral hairy leukoplakia is more predominantly seen in:
    a. Smokers
    b. HSV infected individuals
    c. HIV infected individuals
    d. Individuals exposed to caustic chemicals

54. The causative agent implicated in the etiology of oral hairy leukoplakia is:
    a. HIV
    b. HSV
    c. EBV
    d. Coxsackievirus

55. Oral hairy leukoplakia mainly affects:
    a. Tongue
    b. Buccal mucosa
    c. Lips
    d. Palate

56. The chracteristic microscopic appearance of homogenous viral nuclear inclusions with a residual rim of normal chromatin is a feature of:
    a. Oral hairy leukoplakia
    b. HSV infection
    c. Leukoplakia
    d. Lichen planus

57. Presence of Epstein Barr virus in oral hairy leukoplakia can be demonstrated by all except:
    a. In situ hybridization
    b. Tzanck smear
    c. Electron microscopy
    d. Polymerase chain reaction (PCR)

58. Which disease is called as the disease of the diseased?
    a. Diabetes mellitus
    b. Congenital heart disease
    c. Candidiasis
    d. Lichen planus

59. The organisms capable of producing endogenous cellular nitrosamine production in some strains are:
    a. Candida
    b. Staphylococcus
    c. Rickettsiae
    d. Actinomyces

60. What is the usual concentration of candida in healthy saliva?
    a. 2-5 cells/ml
    b. 20-50 cells/ml
    c. 200-500cells/ml
    d. 2000-5000 cells/ml

Ans. 53. d 54. c 55. a 56. a 57. b 58. c 59. a 60. c

61. Homogenous viral nuclear inclusions are seen in:
    a. Heck's disease
    b. Paget's disease
    c. Oral hairy leukoplakia
    d. White sponge nevus

62. Oral hairy leukoplakia may be associated with all, except:
    a. HIV infection
    b. Prolonged steroid therapy
    c. After organ transplantation
    d. Antihypertensive drug therapy

63. Ephelis refers to:
    a. Increased melanin synthesis by basal layer melanocytes
    b. Gingival enlargement in children
    c. Palatal papillary hyperplasia
    d. Focal epithelial hyperplasia

64. How is grading of oral submucous fibrosis done?

    In the clinical course of oral submucous fibrosis (OSMF), three stages have been identified. These are:
    - Stage of stomatitis and vesiculation
    - Stage of fibrosis
    - Stage of sequelae

    Difficulty in opening the mouth associated with OSMF is graded as given below:
    - < 20 mm : Severe
    - 20-40 mm : Moderate
    - > 40 mm : Mild

    According to the clinical appearance of the lesion, OSMF is graded as given below:

    Grade I: Only blanching of oral mucosa without any symptoms
    Grade II: Burning sensation, dryness of mouth, vesicles or ulcers
    Grade III: In addition to Grade II, restriction of mouth opening
    Grade IV: In addition to Grade III, palpable fibrotic bands all over the mouth without involvement of the tongue
    Grade V: Grade IV and involvement of the tongue
    Grade VI: OSMF with histologically proven oral cancer

65. What are the clinical features of oral submucous fibrosis?

    The following are the clinical features of oral submucous fibrosis?
    - Burning sensation of the mouth

Ans. 61. c 62. a 63. a

- Blanching of oral mucosa
- Atrophy of lingual papillae
- Restriction of mouth opening
- Loss of elasticity of the oral mucosa
- Presence of vertical fibrotic bands
- Sometimes vesicles and bullae
- Ear pain due to involvement of Eustachian tube
- Throat pain due to involvement of pharyngeal mucosa

66. What are the treatment methods available for oral submucous fibrosis?

    The following are the various treatment modalities available for the treatment of oral submucous fibrosis:

    - Avoidance of spicy food
    - Application of topical anesthetizing preparations
    - Intralesional injection of steroids
    - Intralesional injection of collagenolytic agents such as hyaluronidase and placentrix
    - Vitamin supplements
    - Excision of fibrotic bands in severe cases with restricted mouth opening

67. "Hair-on-end" appearance on radiographic examination may be a feature of:

    a. Pernicious anemia
    b. Aplastic anemia
    c. Thalassemia
    d. Aplastic anemia

68. Among the following investigations for the diagnosis of thalassemia, which is incorrect?

    a. Target cell formation and basophilic stippling of erythrocytes
    b. Hypochromic anemia with anisocytosis and poikilocytosis
    c. Lowered total iron-binding capacity (TIBC)
    d. Increase in fetal hemoglobin (HbF)

69. Glucose-6-phosphate dehydrogenase deficiency is:

    a. A clotting Factor abnormality
    b. An intracorpuscular defect of erythrocytes
    c. Abnormal platelet activity
    d. A myeloproliferative disease

Ans. 67. c 68. c 69. b

70. Among the following, which is a condition associated with reduced life span of erythrocytes?
    a. Glucose-6-phosphate-dehydrogenase deficiency
    b. Aplastic anemia
    c. Pernicious anemia
    d. Folic acid deficiency anemia

71. In glucose-6-phosphate-dehydrogenase deficiency which is deficient?
    a. Hemoglobin
    b. Iron
    c. Protein
    d. Glutathione

72. Nitroblue tetrazolium reduction test is:
    a. Caries activity test
    b. Assessment of functioning of WBCs
    c. Test for AIDS
    d. Test for tuberculosis

73. What is leukemoid reaction?
    a. Allergic reaction associated with intake of drugs for leukemia
    b. Persistent neutrophilic count above 30,000/mm^3
    c. Skin lesion associated with leukemia
    d. Stomatitis associated with leukemia

74. Among the following which may not be associated with leukopenia?
    a. Felty's syndrome
    b. SLE
    c. AIDS
    d. Sarcoidosis

75. Among the following, which drug may not be associated with causing leukopenia?
    a. Phenylbutazone
    b. Sulphonamides
    c. Erythromycin
    d. Chloramphenicol

76. The white lace-like pattern seen in case of lichen planus is called:
    a. Chancre
    b. Koebner's phenomenon
    c. Wickham's striae
    d. Id reaction

77. Occurrence of lichen planus, hypertension and diabetes mellitus is called:
    a. Gorlin-Goltz syndrome
    b. Christ-Siemens-Touraine syndrome
    c. Grinspan's syndrome
    d. Melkersson-Rosenthal syndrome

Ans. 70. a 71. d 72. b 73. b 74. d 75. c 76. c 77. c

78. Among the following drugs, which is used in the treatment of leukoplakia?
   a. Vitamin A
   b. Antibiotics
   c. Methotrexate
   d. Steroids

79. Keratotic lesions differ from non-keratotic lesions in that:
   a. It is scrapable
   b. It is non-scrapable
   c. Always turn malignant
   d. No chances for turning malignant

80. The most probable cause for geographic tongue is:
   a. Allergy and emotional stress
   b. Menopause
   c. Viral infection
   d. Bacterial infection

81. Lesion similar to geographic tongue is seen in:
   a. Oral candidiasis
   b. Leukoplakia
   c. Reiter's syndrome
   d. Wegener's granulomatosis

82. Among the following, which is not a feature of pachyonychia congenita?
   a. Thickening of nails
   b. Corneal dystrophy
   c. Fissured tongue
   d. Keratotic thickening of palms and soles

83. Heck's disease is most probably seen in:
   a. Asians
   b. Eskimos
   c. Mongloids
   d. Blacks

84. Nodular acanthosis and subepithelial lymphocyte infiltration are features of:
   a. Focal epithelial hyperplasia
   b. Stomatitis nicotina palatinae
   c. Traumatic keratosis
   d. White sponge nevus

85. Bleeding tendency in case of rheumatoid arthritis may be due to:
   a. Anemia
   b. Thrombocytopenia
   c. Aspirin therapy
   d. Granuloma

Ans. 78. a 79. b 80. a 81. c 82. c 83. b 84. a 85. c

86. Among the following, which is not a laboratory finding of rheumatoid arthritis?
    a. Positive RF
    b. Increased ESR
    c. Macrocytic anemia
    d. Normocytic anemia

87. One of the features not associated with rheumatoid arthritis is:
    a. Subcutaneous nodules
    b. Granuloma
    c. Enlargement of lymph nodes
    d. Microabscess formation

88. The reddish spots seen in case of stomatitis nicotina palatinae are due to:
    a. Inflammation of sebaceous glands
    b. Inflammation of palatal mucosa
    c. Inflamed minor salivary gland openings
    d. Hemorrhagic spots

89. Infection of the fingers by herpes virus is called?
    a. Chancre
    b. Whitlows
    c. Id reaction
    d. Split papules

90. Herpes simplex virus is composed of four layers. These layers are the following:
    - Inner core of linear double-stranded DNA
    - A protein capsid
    - A tegument
    - Lipid envelope containing glycoproteins derived from the nuclear membrane of host cells

91. Herpes simplex virus is composed of how many layers?
    a. One
    b. Two
    c. Three
    d. Four

92. Roseola infantum is caused by:
    a. Epstein-Barr virus
    b. Human herpes virus
    c. Cytomegalovirus
    d. Varicella-zoster virus

Ans. 86. c 87. a 88. c 89. b 91. d 92. b

93. Petechiae are:
   a. Purpuric lesions less than 2 mm
   b. Purpuric lesions more than 2 mm
   c. Raised lesion containing purulent material
   d. Solid raised lesion

94. What is a Tzanck smear?

This refers to the laboratory method used to diagnose herpetic gingivostomatitis. In this study, a fresh vesicle is opened and a scraping is made from the base of the lesion and placed on a microscopic slide. The slide is then stained with Giemsa, Wright or Papanicolaou's stain. Then it is viewed under the microscope for the presence of multinucleated giant cells, syncytium and ballooning degeneration of the nucleus.

It is found that fluorescent staining of cytology smears is more sensitive (83%) than routine cytology.

Tzanck smear is positive in herpes simplex infection.

95. What are the four components of a clinical problem?

The four components of a clinical problem are SOAP. It is a mnemonic for the following:

- S – Subjective (which indicates chief complaint, symptoms and medical history)
- O – Objective (generalized examination and evaluation of the chief complaint)
- A – Assessment (evaluation and arriving at a diagnosis)
- P – Plan (it refers to the treatment plan)

96. What are the conditions to be considered in a patient with cervical lymphadenopathy?

- Acute bacterial, viral and rickettsial infection (e.g., acute abscess, infectious mononucleosis, cat-scratch disease and mucocutaneos lymph node syndrome)
- Chronic bacterial infections (e.g., syphilis and tuberculosis)
- Leukemia
- Lymphoma
- Metastatic carcinoma
- Allergic reactions
- Sarcoidosis

Ans. 93. b

97. Graded Frey's hairs are used to evaluate which cranial nerve?
    a. I
    b. III
    c. V
    d. VII
98. Among the following statements about primary syphilis which is incorrect?
    a. Occurs at the site of infection
    b. Occurs after 2-4 weeks after inoculation
    c. It appears macular, then becomes popular and ulcerates
    d. Ulcer is very painful
99. The organism responsible for causing syphilis is:
    a. Borrelia vincentii
    b. Treponema pallidum
    c. Mycobacterium leprae
    d. Actinomyces israeli
100. Mucous patches are characteristic features of which stage of syphilis?
    a. Primary
    b. Secondary
    c. Tertiary
    d. Congnital

Ans. 97. c 98. d 99. b 100. b

SECTION III

1. Among the following statements about ossifying fibroma which is false?
   a. It has a clearly defined cortical margin
   b. It most often occurs in the maxilla
   c. It is slow growing
   d. It grows into and fills cavities
2. Among the following statements about fibrous dysplasia which is false?
   a. It has a diffuse margin radiographically
   b. It commonly occurs in the mandible
   c. It is slow growing
   d. It grows endosteally
3. Some of the biochemical changes associated with fibrous dysplasia may be the following except:
   a. Increased serum alkaline phosphatase level
   b. High urinary hydroxyproline
   c. Elevated serum calcium level
   d. Normal phosphate level
4. The most ideal treatment for fibrous dysplasia is:
   a. Radiotherapy
   b. Chemotherapy
   c. Superficial recontouring
   d. Combination of surgery and radiotherapy
5. Among the following which is not a feature of Albright's syndrome?
   a. Polyostotic fibrous dysplasia
   b. Endocrine abnormalities
   c. Pigmentation
   d. Intestinal polyposis

Ans. 1. b 2. b 3. c 4. c 5. d

6. The histologic appearance of melanin-containing epithelial cells lining slitlike spaces and small round cells resembling neuroblasts is suggestive of:
   a. Malignant melanoma
   b. Nevus of Ota
   c. Melanotic neuroectodermal tumour
   d. Melanoplakia
7. The large granular cells of granular cell tumour are the following except:
   a. Muscle cells
   b. Histiocytic cells
   c. Schwann cells
   d. Endothelial cells
8. The most common site of occurrence of granular cell tumour is:
   a. Tongue
   b. Lips
   c. Buccal mucosa
   d. Palate
9. Among the following statements about glomus tumour which is incorrect?
   a. It occurs as a result of proliferation of smooth-muscle pericytic cells of arteriovenous anastamosis
   b. These lesions secrete catecholamines
   c. They occur in the pterygotympanic region
   d. The common site of occurrence is the mouth
10. All of the following may be causes for macroglossia, except:
    a. Lymphangioma
    b. Congenital hypothyroidism
    c. Hurler's syndrome
    d. Hypopituitarism
11. Large lymphangiomas spreading into and distending the neck are called:
    a. Thyroglossal cyst
    b. Cystic hygroma
    c. Branchial cyst
    d. Lymphangiosarcoma

Ans. 6. c 7. d 8. a 9. d 10. d 11. b

12. What are hemangiomas?

Hemangiomas are tumourlike malformations consisting of disorganized masses of endothelium-lined vessels that are filled with blood having communication with major blood vascular system.

The common sites of occurrence of hemangioma are:

- Surface mucosa
- Skin
- Jaws
- Facial bones
- Salivary glands
- Muscles
- Temporomandibular joint

Hemangiomas can have two types of presentations:

- Simple red patches (nevus flammeus, Port-wine stain)
- Birthmarks (nongenetically transmitted embryological mishaps).

Treatment:

- Conventional surgery (often associated with the risk of uncontrollable bleeding)
- Cryosurgery
- Laser surgery
- Injection of sclerosing solution
- Intravascular embolization with plastic spheres
- Radiation (for the purpose of sclerosing the lesion)
- Intralesional injection of corticosteroids especially in case of hemangiomas occurring in children

Syndromes associated with hemangioma (angiomatous syndromes):

- Sturge-Weber syndrome (encephalotrigeminal angiomatosis)
- Maffucci's syndrome
- Von Hippel-Lindau disease (familial syndrome involving hemangioblastoma of the retina and cerebellum, pancreatic and renal cysts, renal adenomas, hepatic hemangiomas and multiple endocrine neoplasia

---

Ans.

13. Among the following hamartomas which one has a greater tendency to undergo malignant transformation?
    a. Neurofibroma
    b. Hemangioma
    c. Lymphangioma
    d. Granular cell tumour
14. Among the following which is not a hamartoma?
    a. Glomus tumour
    b. Lymphangioma
    c. Granular cell tumour of the tongue
    d. Pseudoepitheliomatous hyperplasia
15. Pseudoepitheliomatous hyperplasia may occur in all except:
    a. Granular cell tumour of the tongue
    b. Keratoacanthoma of the lips
    c. Leukoplakia of the tongue
    d. Epulis fissuratum
16. The differentiating features of pseudoepitheliomatous hyperplasia are all the following, except:
    a. Extension of rete pegs into the underlying connective tissue
    b. Prominent keratin pearl formation
    c. Cellular atypia
    d. Neutrophilic infiltration
17. Which is the predominant cell type in pseudosarcomatous fascitis?
    a. Myofibroblast
    b. Osteoblast
    c. Endothelial cell
    d. Nerve cell
18. The most favoured site for giant cell granuloma is:
    a. Maxillary canine region
    b. Mandibular third molar region
    c. Incisors to first molar in the mandible
    d. Midline of the mandible
19. Pseudosarcomatous fascitis affects which type of tissue?
    a. Connective tissue
    b. Vascular tissue
    c. Nerve tissue
    d. Bone tissue
20. Osteoclastoma is otherwise known as:
    a. Paget's disease
    b. Peripheral giant cell granuloma
    c. Fibrous dysplasia
    d. Juvenile periodontitis

Ans. 13. a 14. d 15. c 16. a 17. a 18. c 19. a 20. b

21. Occurrence of palatal papillary hyperplasia is stimulated by:
    a. Pan chewing
    b. Dentures
    c. Reverse smoking
    d. Mouth breathing

22. An inflammatory hyperplasia associated with the periphery of ill-fitting dentures is called:
    a. Epulis
    b. Fibroma
    c. Polyp
    d. Epulis fissuratum

23. Presence of multiple microaneurysms owing to a weakening defect in the adventitial coat of venules is suggestive of:
    a. Lymphangioma
    b. Hereditary hemorrhagic telangiectasia
    c. Idiopathic thrombocytopenic purpura
    d. Vitamin C deficiency

24. Kaposi's sarcoma may be treated with intralesional use of:
    a. Methotrexate
    b. Vincristine
    c. Vinblastine
    d. Bleomycin

25. Microscopically, proliferating spindle cells with mild pleomorphism associated with plump endothelial cells oriented about small lumina is suggestive of:
    a. Kaposi's sarcoma
    b. Sjögren's syndrome
    c. Lymphangioma
    d. Rheumatoid arthritis

26. Kaposi's sarcoma occurs along with:
    a. Herpetic infections
    b. Mumps
    c. Parasitic infections
    d. AIDS

27. Kaposi's sarcoma predominantly occurs in:
    a. Palate
    b. Tongue
    c. Buccal mucosa
    d. Floor of the mouth

28. Kaposi's sarcoma is a:
    a. Bone tumour
    b. Vascular tumour
    c. Salivary gland tumour
    d. Sebaceous gland tumour

Ans. 21. b 22. d 23. b 24. c 25. a 26. d 27. a 28. b

29. Angiosarcomas are best treated with:
    a. Radiotherapy
    b. Surgical excision
    c. Chemotherapy
    d. No treatment is required as it is harmless
30. The most common site of occurrence of angiosarcoma is:
    a. Oral cavity
    b. Abdomen
    c. Eyes
    d. Anywhere in the body
31. Degenerative changes of the adventitia of the venous wall will be presented as:
    a. Varices
    b. Calcification of blood vessels
    c. Proliferation of endothelium
    d. Thrombus
32. Varix refers to:
    a. Dilated arteries
    b. Dilated veins
    c. Dilated salivary duct
    d. Dilated capillaries
33. Argon laser is used to treat:
    a. Port-wine stains
    b. Leukoplakia
    c. Oral submucous fibrosis
    d. Syphilitic mucous patches
34. The sclerosing agent 1% sodium tetradecyl sulfate is administered:
    a. Systemically
    b. Intralesionally
    c. Parenterally
    d. Topically
35. A sclerosing agent used to treat hemangioma is:
    a. Hot water
    b. Absolute alcohol
    c. Sodium thiosulfate
    d. Sodium tetradecyl sulfate
36. A treatment modality advocated for hemangioma is:
    a. Radiotherapy
    b. Laser surgery
    c. Chemotherapy
    d. Curettage
37. Calcification of blood vessels is called:
    a. Rhinolith
    b. Antrolith
    c. Phlebolith
    d. Sialolith

Ans. 29. b 30. d 31. a 32. b 33. a 34. b 35. d 36. b 37. c

38. An examination method used to identify a vascular lesion is:
    a. Scintigraphy
    b. Diascopy
    c. Immunofluorescence studies
    d. FNAC

39. The other name for encephalotrigeminal angiomatosis is:
    a. Sturge-Weber syndome
    b. Rendu-Weber-Osler disease
    c. Idiopathic thrombocytopenic purpura
    d. Peutz-Jeghers syndrome

40. An example for proliferation of vascular channels is:
    a. Thrombasthenia
    b. Ecchymosis
    c. Hemangioma
    d. Bleb

41. The treatment advised for ossifying fibroma is:
    a. Radiotherapy
    b. Surface sculpting
    c. Surgical enucleation
    d. Chemotherapy

42. Histologically, resemblance to reparative granuloma with prominent vascular spaces and evidence of hemorrhage are features of:
    a. Lymphangioma
    b. Hemangioma
    c. Aneurysmal bone cyst
    d. Idiopathic thrombocytopenic purpura

43. Submandibular salivary gland depression is also called as:
    a. Latent bone cyst
    b. Follicular cyst
    c. Odontogenic keratocyst
    d. Primordial cyst

44. A characteristic feature of Stafne's cyst is:
    a. Occurrence above inferior alveolar canal
    b. Occurrence below inferior alveolar canal
    c. Honey comb appearance
    d. Ground glass appearance

45. A treatment modality suggested for aneurysmal bone cyst is:
    a. Injection of sclerosing agents
    b. Curettage of the lesion
    c. Surgical resection
    d. Embolization

Ans. 38. b 39. a 40. c 41. c 42. c 43. a 44. b 45. b

46. One of the consistent features associated with cherubism is:
    a. Submandibular lymphadenopathy
    b. Pigmentation
    c. Blue sclera
    d. Egg shell crackling of bone during palpation

47. Cherubism is inherited as:
    a. Sex-linked trait
    b. Dominant gene
    c. Recessive gene
    d. Not genetic

48. In cherubism:
    a. Serum calcium is elevated and phosphorus is decreased
    b. Serum calcium is decreased and phosphorus is elevated
    c. Serum calcium and phosphorus are within normal limits
    d. Serum calcium and phosphorus are elevated

49. Histologically cherubism resembles:
    a. Benign giant cell granuloma
    b. Fibrous dysplasia
    c. Ossifying fibroma
    d. Aneurysmal bone cyst

50. The prominent eosinophilic perivascular cuffing material noted around capillaries in cherubism is:
    a. Osseous tissue
    b. Degenerated blood vessels
    c. Collagen
    d. Salivary gland tissue

51. Endogenous deposition of gold salts used in the treatment of arthritis can result in:
    a. Auric stomatitis
    b. Acrodynia
    c. Peutz-Jegher's syndrome
    d. Argyria

52. Endogenous pigmentation of silver is called:
    a. Mercurialism
    b. Acrodynia
    c. Argyria
    d. Hemochromatosis

53. Excessive adrenocorticotropic hormone secretion can result in:
    a. Excessive salivation
    b. Buffalo hump
    c. Excessive pigmentation
    d. Heat intolerance

Ans. 46. a 47. b 48. c 49. a 50. c 51. a 52. c 53. c

54. The precursor of melanin is:
 a. Tyrosine b. Iron
 c. Hemoglobin d. Valine

55. Generalized hemosiderine tissue pigmentation is termed:
 a. Sideropenic dysphagia
 b. Hemochromatosis
 c. Hemoglobinemia
 d. Auric stomatitis

56. Among the following which is not a cause for endogenous pigmentation of oral mucosa?
 a. Hemoglobin b. Hemosiderin
 c. Nicotine d. Melanin

57. Among the following pigments which cannot accumulate in developing dentine during odontogenesis?
 a. Bilirubin b. Nicotine
 c. Porphyrine d. Hemosiderine

58. Increased keratinization presents as:
 a. White lesion b. Blue lesion
 c. Yellow lesion d. Ulceration

59. On histologic examination, presence of severely atrophic epithelium with complete loss of rete ridges with hyalinization of lamina propria is suggestive of:
 a. Xeroderma
 b. Systemic lupus erythematosus
 c. Oral submucous fibrosis
 d. Myositis ossificans

60. Stiffening of the oral mucosa is a feature of:
 a. Lichen planus
 b. Syphilis
 c. AIDS
 d. Oral submucous fibrosis

61. Odontogenic keratocyst (OKC) is considered to be same as:
 a. Follicular cyst
 b. Primordial cyst
 c. Eruption cyst
 d. Radicular cyst

Ans. 54. a 55. b 56. c 57. b 58. a 59. c 60. d 61. b

62. Radicular cyst is considered to arise as a result of inflammatory proliferation and cystic degeneration of:
    a. Epithelial cell rests of Malassez
    b. Dental papilla
    c. Reduced enamel epithelium
    d. Hertwig's epithelial root sheath

63. Eruption cyst is a soft tissue analogue of:
    a. Follicular cyst
    b. Radicular cyst
    c. Primordial cyst
    d. Globulomaxillary cyst

64. One of the most likely potentials of follicular cyst is:
    a. Anaplastic transformation
    b. Spontaneous regression
    c. Drifting of adjacent roots without resorption
    d. Origin of plexiform ameloblastoma

65. The follicular cyst is considered to originate from:
    a. Epithelial remnants
    b. Dental lamina
    c. Reduced enamel epithelium
    d. Hertwig's epithelial root sheath

66. The oral disease that is prevalent among the inhabitants of Southeast Asia is:
    a. Lichen planus
    b. Sickle cell disease
    c. Oral submucous fibrosis
    d. AIDS

66. A treatment modality that has been tried for psoriasis and geographic tongue is:
    a. Systemic corticosteroids
    b. Topical antifungal agents
    c. Systemic retinoid
    d. Systemic methotrexate

67. Geographic tongue may be associated with which skin lesion?
    a. Lichen planus
    b. Psoriasis
    c. Scabies
    d. Lupus vulgaris

Ans. 62. a 63. a 64. d 65. c 66. d 67. b

68. Erythema circinata migrans refers to:
   a. Oral lesions of erythema multiforme
   b. Ectopic geographic tongue
   c. Red areas associated with lichen planus
   d. Syphilitic mucous patches

69. Epstein's pearls are:
   a. Projections on the enamel
   b. Rete ridges in squamous cell carcinoma
   c. Odontogenic cysts of dental lamina origin
   d. Surgical scars

70. Among the following statements about Fordyce's granules which is correct?
   a. Can undergo malignant transformation
   b. Does not require any treatment
   c. Can predispose to oral candidiasis
   d. Can occur due to allergic response

71. The most common oral change associated with discoid lupus erythematosus is:
   a. Oral candidiasis
   b. Oral ulcers
   c. Hyperplasia of oral mucosa
   d. Depapillation of tongue

72. What is the malignant potential of oral lesions of lupus erythematosus?

   The malignant transformation of oral lesions of lupus erythematosus is controversial. However, cases of squamous cell carcinoma originating in healing scars of discoid lupus erythematosus has been reported. It is generally believed that the malignant transformation may occur because of radiation and ultraviolet light used in the treatment of lupus erythematosus.

73. Deposition of various immunoglobulins and C3 in a granular band involving the basement membrane zone on immunofluorescent studies is suggestive of:
   a. Oral lupus
   b. Lichen planus
   c. Epidermolysis bullosa
   d. Pemphigus

Ans. 68. b 69. a 70. b 71. b 73. a

74. Histopathological changes of hyperorthokeratosis with keratotic plugs, atrophy of the rete ridges and liquefactive degeneration of the basal cell layer are features of:
    a. Oral lupus
    b. Lichen planus
    c. Epidermolysis bullosa
    d. Pemphigus

75. Discoid lupus erythematosus is predominantly seen in:
    a. 1st and 2nd decades
    b. 3rd and 4th decades
    c. 5th and 6th decades
    d. 7th and 8th decades

76. Lyell's disease is also called as:
    a. Toxic epidermal necrolysis
    b. Geographic tongue
    c. Psoriasis
    d. Syphilis

77. Presence of IgM-staining cytoid bodies are suggestive of:
    a. Leukoplakia
    b. Syphilis
    c. White sponge nevus
    d. Lichen planus

78. Civatte bodies of lichen planus are:
    a. Pyknotic nuclear fragments
    b. Cytoplasmic inclusion bodies
    c. Mitochondria
    d. Shrunken plasma membrane

79. Civatte bodies are seen in:
    a. Squamous cell carcinoma
    b. Leukoplakia
    c. Oral submucous fibrosis (OSMF)
    d. Lichen planus

80. Saw-toothed rete pegs is a feature of:
    a. Leukoplakia
    b. Lichen planus
    c. Oral submucous fibrosis
    d. Syphilis

Ans. 74. a 75. b 76. a 77. d 78. a 79. d 80. b

81. The lesion most likely to resemble desquamative gingivitis is:
 a. Periodontal abscess b. Leukoplakia
 c. Lichen planus d. ANUG

82. The type of lichen planus which is more probable for malignant transformation is:
 a. Reticular b. Erosive
 c. Bullous d. Annular

83. Oral lichen planus is considered to be of —— origin:
 a. Parasitic b. Immunological
 c. Infectious d. Inflammatory

84. Bowen's disease can resemble:
 a. Leukoplakia
 b. Erythroplakia
 c. Papillomatous lesion
 d. All of the above

85. Bowen's disease is:
 a. Tuberculosis caused by bovine animals
 b. Intraepidermal squamous cell carcinoma
 c. Extensive oral candidiasis
 d. Paralysis of the facial muscles

86. What is the percentage of aqueous solution used in toluidine blue staining?
 a. 0.1% b. 1.0%
 c. 10.0% d. 100.0%

87. Which are the lesions to be considered in the differential diagnosis of leukoplakia?

 The following are the lesions to be considered in the differential diagnosis of leukoplakia.

 - Lichen planus
 - Lesions caused by cheek-biting
 - Frictional keratosis
 - Tobacco-induced keratosis
 - Nicotinic stomatitis
 - Leukedema
 - White sponge nevus

Ans. 81. c 82. b 83. b 84. d 85. b 86. b

88. Among the following which is not a feature of dysplasia?
    a. Hyperchromic nuclei
    b. Cellular and nuclear pleomorphism
    c. Premature keratinization of individual cells
    d. Decreased nucleocytoplasmic ratio

89. Leukoplakia involving which anatomic site shows dysplasia more often?
    a. Tongue and floor of the mouth
    b. Lips and buccal mucosa
    c. Palate and buccal mucosa
    d. Tongue and palate

90. Parulis refers to:
    a. Granulation tissue covering intraoral sinus
    b. A fulminant fungal infection
    c. Tumourlike malformation
    d. Parasitic infection

91. Cysts of the maxillary sinus are likely to develop from:
    a. Epithelial lining of the oral mucous membrane
    b. Pseudostratified coulumnar respiratory epithelium
    c. Epithelial remnants
    d. Undifferentiated mesenchymal cells

92. Pidborg's tumour is also called as:
    a. Ameloblastoma
    b. Ameloblastic fibroodontoma
    c. Calcifying epithelial odontogenic tumour
    d. Primary intraalveolar carcinoma

93. Gorlin's cyst is also known as:
    a. Radicular cyst
    b. Globulomaxillary cyst
    c. Primordial cyst
    d. Calcifying epithelial odontogenic cyst

94. Among the following cysts which is capable of occurring as a cyst and less commonly as a solid tumour?
    a. Radicular cyst
    b. Gorlin's cyst
    c. Odontogenic keratocyst
    d. Residual cyst

Ans. 88. d 89. a 90. a 91. b 92. c 93. d 94. b

95. Uni- or miltilocular radiopacity enclosing calcified structures of variable size ("Pepper – and – salt" appearance) is a feature of:
   a. Odontogenic keratocyst
   b. Gorlin's cyst
   c. Pindborg's tumour
   d. Ameloblastoma

96. Radiopacity enclosing calcified structures of variable size is known as which appearance?
   a. Cotton wool
   b. Driven snow
   c. Pepper-and-salt
   d. Cumulus cloud

97. Ameloblastoma is best treated by:
   a. Enucleation
   b. Marsupialization
   c. Decompression
   d. Block excision

98. Adenoameloblastoma is an old term for:
   a. Adenomatoid odontogenic tumour
   b. Adenocystic carçinoma
   c. Melanotic neuroectodermal tumour of infancy
   d. Ameloblastic fibroma

99. Melanotic neuroectodermal tumour of infancy is also sometimes called as:
   a. Malignant melanoma
   b. Melanoblastoma
   c. Melanotic ameloblastoma
   d. Melanoblastic fibroma

100. Among the following statements about ameloblastoma which is incorrect?
   a. It is locally invasive
   b. Does not metastasize
   c. Usually occurs in children
   d. Most of the lesions occur in the mandible

Ans. 95. b 96. c 97. d 98. a 99. c 100. c

SECTION IV

1. Microscopically, appearance of fibrous stroma with islands or masses of proliferating epithelium that always resembles the odontogenic epithelium of the enamel organ are features of:
   a. Mucoepidermoid tumour
   b. Ameloblastoma
   c. Pindborg's tumour
   d. Adenomatoid odontogenic tumour

2. Radiotherapy is not indicated for the treatment of ameloblasoma because:
   a. It can cause osteoradionecrosis
   b. It causes anaplastic transformation
   c. It causes radiation-induced sarcoma
   d. It reduces the vascularity of the bone

3. A tumour of odontogenic epithelium with ductlike structure with varying degrees of inductive change in the stroma is a feature of:
   a. Ameloblastoma
   b. Adenomatoid odontogenic tumour
   c. Mucoepidermoid tumour
   d. Osteogenic sarcoma

4. Pindborg's tumour is most likely to resemble:
   a. Ameloblasoma
   b. Adenomatoid odontogenic tumour
   c. Oral squamous cell carcinoma
   d. Osteomyelitis

5. Histologically, masses of polyhedral epithelial cells with little stroma and the cells which are eosinophilic with multiple giant nuclei are features of:
   a. Ameloblastoma
   b. Ameloblastic fibroodontoma
   c. Pindborg tumour
   d. Metastatic carcinoma

Ans. 1. b 2. c 3. a 4. a 5. c

6. The characteristic appearance of hyaline, concentrically calcified globules of amyloid within the masses of epitheloid cells is a feature of:
   a. Ameloblastoma
   b. Ameloblastic fibroodontoma
   c. Pindborg tumour
   d. Metastatic carcinoma
7. Clear cell odontogenic tumour can resemble:
   a. Metastatic tumour
   b. Aneurysmal bone cyst
   c. Pindborg tumour
   d. Condensing osteitis
8. An example for odontogenic tumour of mesenchymal origin is:
   a. Ameloblastoma
   b. Calcifying epithelial odontogenic tumour
   c. Ameloblastic fibroodontoma
   d. Odontogenic myxoma
9. Osteitis fibrosa cystica generalizata is a typical radiographic feature of:
   a. Ameloblastoma
   b. Calcifying epithelial odontogenic tumour
   c. Hyperparathyroidism
   d. Osteoporosis
10. Which tumour is a variant of ossifying fibroma?
   a. Cementifying fibroma
   b. Fibous dysplasia
   c. Paget's disease
   d. Ossifying subperiosteal hematoma
11. The cyst most likely to occur in association with odontoma is:
   a. Radicular cyst
   b. Dentigerous cyst
   c. Globulomaxillary cyst
   d. Primordial cyst
12. An example for virus-induced neoplasm is:
   a. Oral squamous cell carcinoma
   b. Odontogenic myxoma
   c. Squamous papilloma
   d. Ameloblastoma

Ans. 6. c 7. a 8. d 9. c 10. a 11. b 12. c

13. Detection of virus can be done by the following except:
    a. DNA hybridization
    b. Antinuclear antibody test
    c. Restriction endonuclease analysis
    d. Polymerase chain reaction
14. Histologically, presence of nondyskeratotic nodular acanthosis with subepithelial lymphocytic infiltration are features of:
    a. Focal epithelial hyperplasia
    b. Dyskeratosis congenita
    c. Eosinophilic granuloma
    d. Jaw lesions of hyperparathyroidism
15. Among the following, which is not a feature of keratoacanthoma?
    a. It occurs in sun-exposed skin
    b. It undergoes rapid growth
    c. It is not fixed to the surrounding tissue
    d. It is usually capped with thick keratin
16. The finding of six or more macules greater than 1.5 cm in diameter in case of neurofibromatosis is called:
    a. Trousseau's sign
    b. Crowe's sign
    c. Bull's eye sign
    d. Eagle's sign
17. The lesion most likely to demonstrate malignant behaviour is:
    a. Addison's disease
    b. Jaw lesions of hyperparathyroidism
    c. Peutz-Jeghers syndrome
    d. Von Recklinghausen's disease
18. Among the following, which is not a feature of Peutz-Jeghers syndrome?
    a. Polypoid lesions of small intestine
    b. Perioral and lip freckling
    c. Patches brown oral mucosal pigmentation
    d. Endocrine abnormalities
19. Which is the disease associated with jaw cysts, enlarged calvarium and other bony abnormalities such as calcification of meninges and hypoplastic bifid ribs and skin lesions?
    a. Hereditary hypohydrotic ectodermal dysplasia
    b. Nevoid basal cell carcinoma syndrome
    c. Marfan's syndrome
    d. Osteogenesis imperfecta

Ans. 13. b 14. a 15. b 16. b 17. c 18. d 19. b

20. Pitting of the soles and palms is an obvious additional finding of:
    a. Hereditary hypohydrotic ectodermal dysplasia
    b. Nevoid basal cell carcinoma syndrome
    c. Marfan's syndrome
    d. Osteogenesis imperfecta

21. Which is the tumour most likely to occur in association with nevoid basal cell carcinoma syndrome?
    a. Ameloblastoma and fibrosarcoma
    b. Basal cell carcinoma
    c. Papilloma
    d. Squamous cell carcinoma

22. Gastrinoma is the other name of:
    a. Pernicious anemia
    b. Zollinger-Ellison syndrome
    c. Achlorhydria
    d. Aspirin-induced gastric mucosal change

23. Seizures and mental retardation associated with hamartomatous glial proliferation and neuronal deformity in the central nervous system are features of:
    a. Multiple sclerosis
    b. Tuberous sclerosis
    c. Scleroderma
    d. Dermatomyositis

24. Grayish brown thickened patches of skin which are usually symmetrically distributed and which have a characteristic velvety papillosquamous texture are features of:
    a. Acanthosis nigricans
    b. Multiple sclerosis
    c. Tuberous sclerosis
    d. Scleroderma

25. Patients with Albright's syndrome are likely to develop:
    a. Salivary gland tumours
    b. Skin tumours
    c. Bronchogenic carcinoma
    d. Osteosarcoma

Ans. 20. b 21. a 22. b 23. b 24. a 25. d

26. One of the possible etiological factors that is suggested for Paget's disease is:
    a. Bacteria
    b. Virus
    c. Fungus
    d. Endocrine

27. "Leontiasis ossea" is a feature of:
    a. Fibrous dysplasia
    b. Osteogenesis imperfecta
    c. Paget's disease
    d. Hyperparathyroidism

28. The typical radiographic appearance of Paget'd disease is:
    a. Honey comb
    b. Driven snow
    c. Cumulus cloud
    d. Cotton wool

29. One of the antibiotics that is considered to be effective in the management of Paget's disease is:
    a. Kanamycin
    b. Bleomycin
    c. Mithramycin
    d. Sulphonamide

30. What is the action of mithramycin in the treatment of Paget's disease?
    a. Removes secondary infection
    b. Inhibits osteoclastic activity
    c. Reduces bone pain
    d. Reduces alteration of the bone morphology

31. Urinary hydroxyproline levels in Paget's disease is an indicator of:
    a. Carbohydrate metabolism
    b. Protein metabolism
    c. Collagen metabolism
    d. Lipid metabolism

32. Which salt can reduce the bone resorption in case of Paget's disease?
    a. Glucocorticoids
    b. Calcium carbonate
    c. Phosphate
    d. Diphosphonate etidronatc

Ans. 26. b 27. c 28. d 29. c 30. b 31. c 32. d

33. Multiple hamartoma and neoplasia syndrome is also called as:
    a. Cowden's syndrome
    b. MEN syndrome
    c. Rutherford's syndrome
    d. Heerfordt's syndrome

34. "Cobblestone" effect of mucous membrane is a feature of:
    a. Cowden's syndrome
    b. Frictional keratosis
    c. Syphilitic mucous patches
    d. White sponge nevus

35. Occurrence of papillomatous nodules accompanied by lipomas, hemangiomas, neuromas, vitiligo, café-au-lait spots and acromelanosis are features of:
    a. Peutz-Jegher's syndrome
    b. Paterson Kelly syndrome
    c. Cowden's syndrome
    d. Weech's syndrome

36. A syndrome that is associated with increased risk of breast and thyroid carcinomas and gastrointestinal malignancy as well as squamous cell carcinoma of the tongue and basal cell tumours of the perianal skin are features of:
    a. Peutz-Jegher's syndrome
    b. Paterson Kelly syndrome
    c. Cowden's syndrome
    d. Weech's syndrome

37. Localized deposits of lipoprotein is called:
    a. Lipomas
    b. Hurler's syndrome
    c. Xanthomas
    d. Multiple myeloma

38. A familial high-density lipoprotein deficiency inherited as an autosomal recessive condition is called:
    a. Tangier disease
    b. Hurler's syndrome
    c. Multiple myeloma
    d. Amyloidosis

Ans. 33. a 34. a 35. c 36. c 37. c 38. a

39. Among the following which is not a component of Langerhans' cell histiocytosis?
    a. Eosinophilic granuloma
    b. Letterer-Siwe disease
    c. Hand-Schüller-Christian syndrome
    d. Kawasaki disease

40. Among the following which is not a component of Hand-Schüller-Christian syndrome?
    a. Exophthalmos
    b. Diabetes insipidus
    c. Diabetes mellitus
    d. Destructive bone lesions

41. Which cell type proliferates in Langerhans' cell histiocytosis apart from Langerhans' cells?
    a. Macrophages
    b. Neutrophils
    c. Lymphocytes
    d. Fat cells

42. Among the following which is not a type of Langerhans' cell histiocytosis?
    a. Acute disseminated
    b. Chronic disseminated
    c. Acute localized
    d. Chronic localized

43. The treatment method advocated for Langerhans' cell histiocytosis is:
    a. Wide excision
    b. Local curettage
    c. Resection of mandible
    d. No treatment is required as it is self-limiting

44. Jaw bone lesions that contain lipid-filled macrophages rather than Langerhans' cells are usually called:
    a. Giant cell granuloma
    b. Non X histiocytosis
    c. Letterer- Siwe disease
    d. Hyperparathyroidism

Ans. 39. d 40. c 41. a 42. c 43. b 44. b

45. Which is the common site for deposition of amyloid in the oral cavity in case of amyloidosis?
    a. Tongue and gingivae
    b. Tongue and palate
    c. Gingivae and buccal mucosa
    d. Tongue and tonsillar region

46. The concentric calcific concretions seen in the granulomatous response of sarcoid granulomas are called:
    a. Civatte bodies
    b. Colloid bodies
    c. Schaumann's bodies
    d. Lipschutz bodies

47. "Ray fungus" is a term given for:
    a. Clostridium tetani
    b. Candida albicans
    c. Actinomyces israelii
    d. Treponema pallidum

48. Clinically and radiographically, actinomycosis can be confused with:
    a. Tuberculosis
    b. Syphilis
    c. Periapical abscess
    d. Pericoronitis

49. How is Actinomyces israelii demonstrated?
    a. Culture studies
    b. In stained tissue sections
    c. Dark field microscopy
    d. Immunofluorescence studies

50. Actinomycotic granuloma is occasionally identified in:
    a. Buccal mucosa
    b. Tonsillar crypts
    c. Periodontal pockets
    d. Periapical tissues of non-vital teeth

51. Which are the different types of actinomycosis?

    Actinomycosis is an infectious disease caused by a slender gram-positive rod-shaped bacterium, *Actinomyces israelii* which exhibits funguslike characteristics and hence it is called as the "ray fungus".

Ans. 45. a 46. c 47. c 48. a 49. b 50. d

The organism is of low virulence and it elicits suppuration, necrosis and a chronic granulomatous response.

The following are the various types of actinomycosis:

- Cervicofacial actinomycosis
- Pulmonary actinomycosis
- Ileocecal actinomycosis
- Pelvic actinomycosis

52. "Lumpy jaw" in cattle is similar to:

a. Periapical abscess
b. Cellulitis
c. Actinomycosis
d. Tuberculosis

53. The frequent site involved by actinomycosis is:

a. Submental region
b. Submandibular region
c. Parotid region
d. Infratemporal region

54. What is the characteristic feature of actinomycosis?

a. Lack of immediate tissue reaction
b. Presence of intense immediate tissue reaction
c. Infection does not originate from a non-healing socket
d. Origin in the submental region

55. Actinomycosis is best treated with:

a. Corticosteroids
b. Amphotericin B
c. Penicillin
d. Streptomycin

56. The organism considered to be of etiological significance in case of cat-scratch disease is:

a. HSV type I
b. HIV
c. Corynebacterium
d. Rochalimaea henselae

57. Cat-scratch disease is best treated by:

a. Immunosuppressive medication
b. Antibiotics
c. Analgesic and antipyretic agents
d. No treatment is required as it is self-limiting

58. Fernandez or Mitsuda reactions are features of:

a. Hansen's disease
b. Tuberculosis
c. Sarcoidosis
d. Actinomycosis

Ans. 52. c 53. b 54. a 55. c 56. d 57. d 58. a

59. Leonine facies is a feature of:
    a. Hansen's disease
    b. Tuberculosis
    c. Sarcoidosis
    d. Actinomycosis

60. Histologically, granulomatous masses consisting of lipid-rich foamy cells with large numbers of acid-fast bacilli is a feature of:
    a. Syphilis
    b. Tuberculosis
    c. Hansen's disease
    d. Actinomycosis

61. Which form of Hansen's disease is more often associated with oral lesions?
    a. Tuberculoid
    b. Lepromatous
    c. Borderline
    d. Reactional

62. The characteristic oral lesions of lepromatous leprosy are:
    a. Ulcerations
    b. Areas of necrosis
    c. White patches
    d. Nodules

63. Among the following drugs which is not associated with enlargement of the gingiva?
    a. Anticonvulsants
    b. Calcium channel blockers
    c. Immunosuppressive medications
    d. Antiallergic agents

64. Scorbutic gingivitis is associated with deficiency of which vitamin?
    a. A
    b. B
    c. C
    d. D

65. Among mouth breathers, gingival inflammation is usually seen in:
    a. Maxillary anterior region
    b. Maxillary posterior region
    c. Mandibular anterior region
    d. Mandibular posterior region

66. Phenytoin-induced gingival hyperplasia is usually seen following intake of the drug more than:
    a. 3 days
    b. 3 weeks
    c. 3 months
    d. 3 years

Ans. 59. a 60. c 61. b 62. d 63. d 64. c 65. a 66. c

67. Topical and systemic use of which drug has been found to be beneficial in case of phenytoin-induced gingival hyperplasia?
    a. Analgesics
    b. Antibiotics
    c. Folic acid
    d. Vitamin C

68. Phenytoin administered during pregnancy can cause:
    a. Neonatal jaundice
    b. Enamel hypoplasia
    c. Gingival hyperplasia during childhood
    d. Congenital anomalies

69. Among the following syndromes which is not associated with gingival enlargement?
    a. Rutherford
    b. Zimmerman-Laband
    c. Gorlin-Goltz
    d. Nezelopf's

70. Among the following which is not a feature of Rutherford's syndrome?
    a. Epiphora
    b. Enlargement of gingiva
    c. Delayed tooth eruption
    d. Superior corneal opacities

71. Among the following which is not a feature of Zimmerman-Laband syndrome?
    a. Gingival fibromatosis
    b. Ear, nose, bone and nail defects
    c. "Froglike" fingers and toes
    d. Angiomatosis

72. Among the following which is not a feature of tuberous sclerosis?
    a. Fibromas of the gingivae
    b. Facial edema
    c. Adenoma sebaceum
    d. Fibromas of the oral mucosa

73. Among the following which is not a feature of Cross syndrome?
    a. Gingival and alveolar enlargement
    b. Microphthalmia
    c. Facial paralysis
    d. Athetosis

Ans. 67. c 68. d 69. d 70. a 71. d 72. b 73. c

74. Among the following which is not a feature of Ramon syndrome?

a. Gingival fibromatosis
b. Hypertrichosis
c. Mental retardation
d. Oral ulcerations

75. Which are the carcinogens present in tobacco?

Tobacco contains the following potent carcinogens:

- Nitrosamines (nicotine)
- Polycyclic aromatic hydrocarbons
- Nitrosodichanolamine
- Nitrosoproline
- Polonium

Tobacco smoke contains the following?

- Carbon monoxide
- Thiocyanate
- Hydrogen cyanide
- Nicotine
- Metabolites of the above constituents

76. What is TNM classification of tumours of the oral cavity?

Tumour, node, metastasis (TNM) system of cancer classification was proposed by the American Joint Committee on cancer (AJCC).

T (Size of Primary Tumour):

Tis: Carcinoma in situ

T1: Tumour less than 2 cm

T2: Tumour more than 2 cm and less than 4 cm

T3: Tumour more than 4 cm

T4: Tumour more than 4 cm with invasion of adjacent structures (ie., through cortical bone; deep into extrinsic muscles of tongue, maxillary sinus and skin)

N (Cervical Lymph Node Metastasis):

N0: No node involvement detected

N1: Single ipsilateral node less than 3 cm

N2a: Single ipsilateral node less than 6 cm

N2b: Multiple ipsilateral nodes more than 3 cm and less than 6 cm

N2c: Bilateral or contralateral lymph nodes less than 6 cm

N3a: Ipsilateral node more than 6 cm

N3b: Bilateral nodes more than 6 cm

M (Distant Metastases):

M0: No known metastases

M1: Metastases present

Ans. 74. d

77. What is TNM staging?
    Stage 1: T1N0M0
    Stage 2: T2N0M0
    Stage3: T3N0M0; T1,T2, or T3N1M0
    Stage 4: T4 any N M0; any TN2 or N3M0; any T or N, with M1

78. What is the classification and staging of oral leukoplakia?
    Provisional (clinical) diagnosis
    L: Extent of leukoplakia
    L0, no evidence of lesion
    L1, less than 2cm
    L2, 2-4 cm
    L3, more than 4 cm
    Lx, not specified
    S: Site of leukoplakia
    S1, all sites excluding floor of mouth and/or tongue
    S2, Floor of mouth and/or tongue
    Sx, not specified
    C: Clinical aspect
    C1, homogenous
    C2, nonhomogenous
    Cx, not specified
    Definitive (histopathologic) diagnosis
    P: histopathologic features
    P1, no dysplasia
    P2, mild dysplasia
    P3, Moderate dysplasia
    P4, Severe dysplasia
    Px, not specified
    Staging
    1: any L, S1, C1, P1 or P2
    2: any L, S1 or S2, C2, P1 or P2
    3: any L, S2, C2, P1 or P2
    4: any L, any S, any C, P3 or P4

79. False positive test result with toluidine blue staining can occur in case of:

    a. Carcinoma in situ
    b. Malignancy
    c. Inflammatory areas
    d. Leukoplakia

Ans. 79. c

80. Computer-assisted analysis of oral brush cytology helps to identify:
    a. Oral candidiasis
    b. AIDS
    c. Oral submucous fibrosis
    d. Abnormal cell morphology and keratinization

81. Statsistically what is the percentage of dysplastic changes to occur in case of leukoplakia?
    a. 90-100
    b. 50-70
    c. 20-30
    d. 2-25

82. Which virus is associated with the etiology of proliferative verrucous leukoplakia (PVL)?
    a. Human papillomavirus
    b. HSV
    c. HIV
    d. Epstein- Barr

83. Which is the common associated infection seen in case of leukoplakia?
    a. Streptococcus infection
    b. Staphylococcus infection
    c. Actinomycosis
    d. Candidiasis

84. Use of smokeless tobacco is associated with:
    a. Reduced incidence of leukoplakia
    b. Increased incidence of leukoplakia
    c. No effect in inducing leukoplakia
    d. None of the above

85. An example for immunologically mediated mucocutaneous disease is:
    a. Lichen planus
    b. Aphthous ulcer
    c. Candidiasis
    d. Oral submucous fibrosis

86. Statistically, what is the percentage of transformation of lichen planus into malignancy?
    a. 75-100
    b. 42-50
    c. 2-18
    d. 0.4-2.5

Ans. 80. d 81. d 82. a 83. d 84. b 85. d 86. d

87. Among the following statements about oral submucous fibrosis which is wrong?
    a. There is epithelial atrophy
    b. There is fibrosis of the submucosa
    c. There is epithelial metaplasia
    d. There is juxtaepithelial inflammatory reaction
88. Among the following statements about oral hairy leukoplakia which is correct:
    a. It is mainly seen among smokers
    b. It is associated with leukoplakia
    c. It is seen in patients with chronic immunosuppression
    d. It is seen in patients who wear dentures
89. Laser excision/ablation of leukoplakia is done with which laser?
    a. Carbon dioxide
    b. Carbon tetrachloride
    c. Ethylene dioxide
    d. Ethylene bisulphide
90. Mild dysplastic cases of leukoplakia can be managed with topical application of:
    a. Vitamin A
    b. Vitamin B
    c. Vitamin C
    d. Vitamin E
91. Which vitamin is supposed to have a significant beneficial role in oral cancer?
    a. A
    b. B
    c. C
    d. D
92. A positive correlation has been proposed between fluoride and—
    a. Oral sqamous cell carcinoma
    b. Osteosarcoma
    c. Bronchogenic carcinoma
    d. Parotid salivary gland tumour
93. Which is the best diagnostic modality that is available for the detection of bone involvement in case of oral squamous cell carcinoma?
    a. Routine extraoral radiographs
    b. Intraoral periapical radiograph
    c. Bone scanning
    d. Fluoroscopy

Ans. 87. c 88. c 89. a 90. a 91. a 92. b 93. c

94. Among the following, which is not an effective diagnostic modality to study involvement of bone by oral cancer:
    a. Bone scanning
    b. Conventional radiographs
    c. Magnetic resonance imaging (MRI)
    d. Fluoroscopy

95. Advanced cases of lung involvement due to metastasis of oral cancer can be identified by:
    a. Fluoroscopy
    b. Conventional radiography
    c. Bone scan
    d. Magnetic resonance imaging

96. Among the following features about dysplasia, which is incorrect?
    a. Increased mitotic figures
    b. Hypochromatism
    c. Nuclear pleomorphism
    d. Alteration in normal cellular orientation

97. Fine needle aspiration cytology is a useful diagnostic aid in case of:
    a. Aphthous ulcers
    b. Oral submucous fibrosis
    c. Oral cancer
    d. Parotid tumour

98. Among the following statements about poorly differentiated carcinoma, which is incorrect?
    a. Do not retain anatomic features of epithelial cells
    b. Do not retain the function of cells
    c. Produce keratin
    d. None of the above

99. In order to recognize tumour invasion, which is the most reliable diagnostic modality?
    a. Immunocytochemistry
    b. Study of lymphatics
    c. Evaluation of blood vessels
    d. Study of perineural spaces

Ans. 94. c 95. b 96. b 97. d 98. c 99. a

100. What are the factors influenzing the treatment of oral cancer?

There are various factors to be considered in the treatment of oral cancer. These factors are the following:

- Cell type
- Degree of differentiation
- Site of the lesion
- Size of the lesion
- Location of the primary lesion
- Lymph node status
- The presence of bone involvement
- The feasibility of obtaining adequate surgical margins
- The ability to preserve functions such as speech, swallowing etc.
- Physical and mental status of the patient
- A deep assessment of the potential complications of each therapy
- Expertise of the surgeon as well as the radiotherapist
- Personal preference of the medical team that manages the patient
- Co-operation of the patient
- Age of the patient

Ans.

SECTION V

1. What are the indications for surgical treatment of oral cancer?

   The following are the indications for surgical treatment of oral cancer.

   - As part of the combined treatment
   - Tumours involving bone
   - When the side effects of surgery are less than that of radiotherapy
   - No significant cosmetic deformity is associated with surgery
   - For tumours that are not sensitive to radiation
   - For recurrent tumours in areas that have received a high radiation dose
   - For palliative purpose
   - To reduce the bulk of the tumour and to enhance the function

2. What are the factors associated with biologic effect of radiation?

   The biologic effects of radiation are dependent on the following factors:

   - Dose per fraction
   - The number of fractions per day
   - The total treatment time
   - The total dose of radiation

3. Brachytherapy is indicated in the following cases except:

   a. Tumours in the posterior aspect of the oral cavity
   b. For localized tumours
   c. For boosted doses of radiation to a specific site
   d. Treatment of recurrences

4. Among the following, which is not an isotope used in brachytherapy?

   a. Cesium b. Helium
   c. Iridium d. Gold

Ans. 3. a 4. b

5. Metastatic tumours of the jaw mainly affect:
   a. Anterior maxilla
   b. Posterior maxilla
   c. Anterior mandible
   d. Posterior mandible

6. The virus implicated in the etiology of nasopharyngeal carcinoma is:
   a. HSV
   b. HIV
   c. Epstein-Barr
   d. Cytomegalovirus

7. The most probable etiological factor associated with the etiology of basal cell carcinoma is:
   a. Virus
   b. Chemicals
   c. Infection
   d. Sunlight

8. Among the following statements about malignant melanoma, which is incorrect?
   a. It is extremely rare
   b. Oral lesions can present as masses or ulcers
   c. It is an aggressive malignant disease
   d. Most of the lesions present on the floor of the mouth

9. Which is the common sarcoma that occurs in the head and region?
   a. Rhabdomyosarcoma
   b. Chondrosarcoma
   c. Osteosarcoma
   d. Fibrosarcoma

10. Which is the commonest tumour associated with HIV infection?
    a. Rhabdomyosarcoma
    b. Oral squamous cell carcinoma
    c. Pleomorphic adenoma
    d. Lymphoma

11. Which is the most rapidly increasing tumour?
    a. Lymphoma
    b. Oral squamous cell carcinoma
    c. Pleomorphic adenoma
    d. Rhabdomyosarcoma

Ans. 5. d 6. c 7. d 8. d 9. a 10. d 11. a

12. What are the essential oral and dental assessment that has to be done prior to cancer treatment?

    The following are the assessment measures that have to be carried out prior to cancer treatment:

    - Reduce the risk of severity of complications
    - Reduce the risk of infection involving dentition and mucosa
    - Minimize complications associated with hyposalivation or xerostomia
    - Extraction of non-restorable teeth
    - Caries prevention programmes, for maintenance of oral hygiene as well as fluoride application
    - Shielding of intraoral areas to avoid unnecessary radiation exposure
    - Planning rehabilitation programmes

13. What are the complications associated with radiotherapy?

    Radiotherapy is associated with the following complications:

    - Direct tissue toxicity
    - Radiation mucositis
    - Secondary bacterial infection
    - Hypovascularity
    - Decreased healing capacity
    - Fibrosis of connective tissue and muscles
    - Epithelial atrophy
    - Altered vascular supply
    - Atrophic and friable mucosa
    - Fibrosis in joint tissue
    - Loss of acinar cells of the salivary glands
    - Alteration in the duct epithelium
    - Fibrosis of salivary gland
    - Fatty degeneration of the salivary gland
    - Increased risk of developing osteoradionecrosis

14. Plasma glutamyl-cysteinyl-glycine (GSH) level is an indicator of severity of:

    a. Radiation mucositis
    b. Oral submucous fibrosis
    c. Addison's disease
    d. Jaundice

Ans. 14. a

15. Among the following, which is associated with promotion of repair of damaged DNA and scavenging of free radicals generated in tissues exposed to radiation?
    a. Corticosteroids
    b. Alpha 1- antitrypsin
    c. Amifostine (Ethyol)
    d. Zinc peroxide

16. Administration of pilocarpine has been found to be effective in:
    a. Xerostomia
    b. Ptyalism
    c. Stomatitis
    d. Mucositis

17. Hyperbaric oxygen (HBO) therapy has been found to be useful in case of:
    a. Oral submucous fibrosis
    b. Osteomyelitis
    c. Rampant caries
    d. Osteoradionecrosis

18. Wharton's duct refers to:
    a. Parotid salivary gland duct
    b. Submandibular salivary gland duct
    c. Sublingual salivary gland duct
    d. Minor salivary gland duct

19. The acinar cells of the parotid gland are:
    a. Serous
    b. Mucous
    c. Mostly serous and to a lesser extent mucous
    d. Mostly mucous and to a lesser extent serous

20. Sialosis refers to:
    a. Excessive salivation
    b. Noninflammatory nonneoplastic enlargement of salivary gland
    c. Difficulty in swallowing
    d. Difficulty in speech

21. Stenson's duct refers to the duct of which salivary gland?
    a. Parotid
    b. Submandibular
    c. Sublingual
    d. Accessory

Ans. 15. c 16. a 17. d 18. b 19. a 20. b 21. a

22. Saliva secretion is stimulated by:
    a. Sympathetic neural input
    b. Parasympathetic neural input
    c. Both sympathetic and parasympathetic input
    d. Independent of sympathetic and parasympathetic input

23. Stimulation for protein release for saliva secretion is by:
    a. Muscarinic cholinergic receptors
    b. Beta-adrenergic receptors
    c. Both muscarinic and beta-adrenergic receptors
    d. Independent of both cholinergic and beta-adrenergic receptors

24. Among the following which is the action of muscarinic agonists?
    a. The salivary gland to transport fluid and to produce saliva
    b. To block transport of fluid and production of saliva
    c. For effective taste perception
    d. To enhance protein production by the salivary gland

25. What is rexostomia?

    Xerostomia refers to dryness of the mouth. The major cause for xerostomia is salivary gland dysfunction. However, it must be emphasized that apart from salivary gland dysfunction there are various other causes also. These causes are listed below :

    Causes:

    - Salivary gland dysfunction
    - Atresia of salivary gland
    - Hypoplasia of the salivary gland
    - Obstruction due to calculi
    - Dehydration
    - Central cognitive alterations and oral sensory disturbances
    - Psychological conditions such as stress and anxiety
    - Radiation therapy
    - Drug-induced (e.g., tricyclic antidepressants)

    Symptoms:

    - Dryness of the mouth including the throat
    - Difficulty in chewing, swallowing and speaking
    - Decreased taste perception
    - Inability to swallow dry foods
    - Frequent sipping of water
    - Mucosal sensitivity to spicy and course food

Ans. 22. c 23. b 24. a

Clinical features:

- Signs of obvious mucosal dryness
- Cracking, peeling and atrophic changes of the lips
- Buccal mucosa may appear pale and corrugated
- Tongue appears smooth and reddened
- Atrophy of lingual papillae
- Sticking of lips to the teeth
- Increased incidence of erosion and dental caries
- Susceptibility for oral candidiasis
- Enlargement of salivary gland

Investigations:

- Salivary flow rate
- Plain-film radiography
- Sialography
- Ultrasonography
- Radionuclide salivary imaging
- Computed tomography and magnetic resonance imaging
- Salivary gland biopsy

Treatment:

- Identification of the cause and correction of the same
- Artificial saliva substitutes
- Frequent sipping of water
- Use of commercially available mouth-wetting agents
- Salivary gland stimulation

26. Carlson-Crittenden collectors are used for collection of:

    a. Urine b. Saliva
    c. Crevicular fluid d. Pus

27. Unstimulated whole saliva flow rate below which level is considered to be abnormal?

    a. 0.01 ml b. 0.1 ml
    c. 1.0 ml d. 10.0 ml

28. A contraindication for performing sialography is:

    a. Neoplasm
    b. Active infection
    c. Obstruction
    d. Presence of mucosal plugs

Ans. 26. b 27. b 28. b

29. The normal salivary gland appearance on a sialogram is described as:
    a. Leafless tree appearance
    b. Branchless fruit-laden appearance
    c. Ball-in-hand appearance
    d. Cherry blossom appearance

30. Sialectasis refers to:
    a. Enlargement of salivary gland
    b. Tumour involving the salivary gland
    c. Stasis of the saliva flow
    d. Appearance of focal collection of contrast medium in sialography

31. Punctate, globular and cavitary sialectasis are descriptive of:
    a. Types of salivary gland neoplasms
    b. Stages of salivary gland aplasia
    c. Progression of severity of sialectasis
    d. Salivary gland appearance after surgical removal of the salivary glands

32. Biopsy of which salivary gland is useful in the evaluation of Sjögren's syndrome?
    a. Parotid
    b. Submandibular
    c. Sublingual
    d. Minor salivary glands

33. Which is the favourite site of accessory mucous gland biopsy to evaluate Sjögren's syndrome?
    a. Labial
    b. Buucal
    c. Lingual
    d. Palatal

34. Among the following, which is a test that can be used to diagnose amyloidosis?
    a. Serum calcium level
    b. Serum alkaline phosphatase level
    c. Minor salivary gland biopsy
    d. Growth hormone studies

35. Immunophenotyping is a useful study of minor salivary glands in the diagnosis of:
    a. Lichen planus
    b. Aphthous ulcers
    c. Lymphoma
    d. Squamous cell carcinoma

Ans. 29. a 30. d 31. c 32. d 33. a 34. c 35. c

36. Serological investigations such as the following except —— may be helpful in the diagnosis of xerostomia:
    a. Antinuclear antibodies
    b. Rheumatoid factors
    c. Elevated immunoglobulins
    d. Vanillylmandelic assay

37. A serologic marker that can be used in the evaluation of salivary gland disorders is:
    a. Ascorbic acid
    b. Amylase
    c. Calcium
    d. Alkaline phosphatase

38. Determination of amylase isoenzymes is done of which tissue to evaluate salivary gland disorder?
    a. Pancreatic and salivary
    b. Renal and pancreatic
    c. Gastric and renal
    d. Intestinal and pancreatic

39. Cystic lymhoepithelial lesions are often associated with which disease?
    a. HIV infection
    b. HSV infection
    c. Periapical abscess
    d. MEN syndrome

40. Fine needle aspiration (FNA) study is basically of:
    a. Blood vessels
    b. Muscles
    c. Joints
    d. Individual cells

41. Malformation of the first branchial arch is often associated with:
    a. Enamel hypoplasia
    b. Dentinogenesis imperfecta
    c. Absence of salivary gland
    d. Absence of mandible

42. Among the following conditions which is not associated with parotid gland agenesis?
    a. Hemifacial microstomia
    b. Mandibulofacial dysostosis
    c. Ectodermal dysplasia
    d. Lacrimoauriculodentodigital syndrome

Ans. 36. d 37. b 38. a 39. a 40. d 41. c 42. c

43. Aberrant salivary glands refer to:
    a. Salivary glands developing at unusual anatomic sites
    b. Absence of salivary glands
    c. Hypoplasia of salivary gland
    d. Atrophic changes of the salivary gland

44. Staphne's cyst refers to:
    a. Salivary gland resting within the depression on the lingual aspect of posterior mandible
    b. Pseudocyst occurring within the body of the mandible due to hemorrhage
    c. Mucous retention cyst occurring in the maxillary antrrum
    d. An inflammatory cyst occurring due to severe infection

45. Diverticuli of the salivary gland refer to:
    a. Intraglandular neoplasms
    b. Outpouching of the duct
    c. Occurrence of salivary glands in unusual locations
    d. Calculi within the salivary gland duct

46. Salivary duct abnormalities may be a feature of:
    a. Ectodermal dysplasia
    b. Staphne's cyst
    c. Darier's disease
    d. Heck's disease

47. What is sialolithiasis?

Sialolithiasis refers to calcified and organic matter that form within the secretory system of the major salivary glands. The exact cause is not known. It may be associated with the following causes:

- Inflammation
- Irregularities in the duct pattern
- Local irritants
- Anticholinergic medications causing pooling of saliva within the duct
- Chronic trauma. Altered salivary hydrogen ion concentration
- Abnormal serum calcium and phosphorus level

Composition:

The structure of sialoliths is crystalline and it is mainly composed of hydroxyapatite. The chemical constituents are the following:

- Calcium

Ans. 43. a 44. a 45. b 46. c

- Phosphate
- Carbon
- Magnesium
- Potassium chloride
- Ammonium

Site:

The common site of occurrence is the submandibular gland. The reasons suggested for occurrence of sialolithiasis in the submandibular gland may be the following:

- The relatively tortuous course of Wharton's duct
- Higher calcium and phosphate levels
- More viscous nature
- Drainage is against the gravity

Clinical features:

- Patients often present history of acute, painful and intermittent swelling of the affected major salivary gland
- The pain is experienced before eating food
- The involved gland is enlarged and tender
- Stasis of saliva can lead to infection, fibrosis and atrophy of the gland
- In chronic cases there can be fistula formation, sinus tract formation and ulceration
- Severe inflammation of the adjacent soft tissue
- Predisposition to sialadenitis, ductal stricture and ductal dilatation

Investigations:

- Radiographic examination, especially mandibular occlusal radiograph
- Sialography
- CT
- FNA studies
- Ultrasonography

Treatment:

- Acute phase is managed with analgesics and antipyretics, rehydration and antibiotics
- Surgical intervention for drainage

Ans.

- Stones near the ductal opening can be removed by milking procedure
- Surgical excision
- Lithotrypsy (extracortical lithotrypsy)

48. Ranula refers to:
    a. An inflammatory cyst occurring within the lining of maxillary sinus
    b. A mucocele occurring in the floor of the mouth
    c. A cyst affecting the minor salivary glands of the palate
    d. Ectopic salivary gland

49. Necrotizing sialometaplasia refers to:
    a. Neoplasm affecting pharyngeal mucosa
    b. A malignant salivary gland tumour
    c. Reactive inflammatory disorder
    d. A complication of acute necrotizing sialometaplasia

50. Necrosis, pseudoepitheliomatous hyperplasia of the mucosal epithelium and squamous metaplasia are features of:
    a. Squamous cell carcinoma
    b. Sjögren's syndrome
    c. Ameloblastoma
    d. Necrotizing sialometaplasia

51. Among the following drugs, which is not implicated in the etiology of allergic sialadenitis?
    a. Phenobarbital
    b. Phenothiazine
    c. Sulfisoxazole
    d. Nimuselide

52. Among the following viruses, which is not implicated in causing salivary gland enlargement?
    a. Paramyxovirus
    b. Coxsackie virus
    c. Cytomegalovirus
    d. Echovirus

53. Mumps is caused by:
    a. Paramyxovirus
    b. Epstein-Barr virus
    c. Cytomegalovirus
    d. Echovirus

Ans. 48. b 49. c 50. d 51. d 52. b 53. a

54. Epidemic parotitis refers to:
    a. Acute suppurative bacterial sialadenitis
    b. Noninflammatory nonneoplastic enlargement of parotid gland
    c. Inflammation involving only the parotid duct
    d. Mumps

55. Among the following statements about mumps, which is incorrect?
    a. It is caused by paramyxovirus
    b. Usually it occurs in children between 4 and 6 years
    c. As yet no vaccine is available to prevent the disease
    d. There is an incubation period lasting 2 to 3 weeks

56. One of the etiological factors proposed in the etiology of autism and inflammatory bowel disease is:
    a. Exposure to radiation
    b. Iron deficiency anemia
    c. Bacterial meningitis
    d. MMR vaccination

57. Mumps generally affects which salivary gland?
    a. Parotid
    b. Submandibular
    c. Sublingual
    d. Accessory

58. Mumps is a disease affecting ——
    a. Sebaceous glands
    b. Lymph nodes
    c. Salivary gland
    d. Lining of the maxillary sinus

59. The incubation period for mumps can range from:
    a. 2-3 days
    b. 2-3 weeks
    c. 2-3 months
    d. 2-3 years

60. A laboratory test to diagnose mumps is:
    a. ELISA test
    b. Immunofluorescence
    c. Antibodies to the S and V antigen
    d. Biopsy
    e. Culture and sensitivity

61. Among the following which is not a complication of mumps?
    a. Encephalitis
    b. Myocarditis
    c. Neuritis
    d. Retinitis

Ans. 54. d 55. c 56. d 57. a 58. c 59. b 60. c 61. d

62. Cytomegalovirus only affects:
    a. Humans
    b. Cattle
    c. Domestic cats
    d. Dogs

63. Cytomegalovirus is responsible for:
    a. Infectious mononucleosis
    b. Hepangina
    c. Hand-foot-and mouth disease
    d. Epidemic parotitis

64. Among the following which is considered as a clinical marker of AIDS?
    a. Herpes simplex infection
    b. Cytomegalovirus infection
    c. Herpangina
    d. Mumps

65. Histological examination of the infected tissue revealing large atypical cells with inclusion bodies which can be two times the normal size with eccentrically placed nuclei, resulting in an "owl-like" appearance is suggestive of:
    a. HSV infection
    b. HIV infection
    c. Systemic lupus erythematosus
    d. Cytomegalovirus infection

66. Past cytomegalovirus infection is identified by:
    a. Culture studies
    b. IgG antibodies against the disease
    c. Saliva analysis
    d. Presence of viral antigen

67. IIIV salivary gland disease (HIV-SGD) mainly affects which salivary glands?
    a. Parotid
    b. Submandibular
    c. Sublingual
    d. Accessory

68. Peripheral blood changes such as hypergammaglobulinemia, circulating immune complexes and rheumatoid factors can be a feature of:
    a. Lichen planus
    b. Sjögren's syndrome
    c. Systemic lupus erythematosus
    d. Scleroderma

Ans. 62. a 63. a 64. b 65. d 66. b 67. a 68. b

69. Hepatitis C virus has recently been implicated in the etiology of:
    a. Sjögren's syndrome
    b. Angioneurotic edema
    c. Nasopharyngeal carcinoma
    d. White sponge nevus

70. The viral infection more likely to cause salivary gland enlargement is:
    a. HSV type I
    b. HSV type II
    c. Hepatitis B virus
    d. Hepatitis C virus

71. "Surgical parotitis " is a name given for:
    a. Epidemic parotitis (mumps)
    b. Bacterial sialadenitis
    c. Allergic parotitis
    d. None of the above

72. The common site of occurrence of bacterial sialadenitis is:
    a. Parotid
    b. Submandibular
    c. Sublingual
    d. Accessory

73. Bacterial sialadenitis occurring in the submandibular gland is very rare because of the following except:
    a. Because of the high level of mucin in the saliva
    b. The particular anatomic location
    c. Tongue movements have a cleansing action
    d. Relatively high acidity of the saliva

74. Which are the systemic conditions associated with salivary gland involvement?

    The following are the various systemic conditions associated with salivary gland involvement:

    - Infections
      Actinomycosis
      Granulomatous diseases such as sarcoidosis and tuberculosis
      HIV-salivary gland disease
      Hepatitis
      Cytomegalovirus infection

Ans. 69. a 70. d 71. b 72. a 73. d

- Metabolic disorders
  Sjögren's syndrome
  Thyroid disease
  Granulomatous disease
  Alcoholism
  Malnutrition
  Eating disorders (anorexia, bulimia)
  Uncontrolled diabetes mellitus
- Neoplasms
  Benign (pleomorphic adenoma, monomorphic adenoma, ductal papilloma)
- Malignant
  Lymphoma
  Mucoepidermoid carcinoma
  Adenoid cystic carcinoma
  Acinic cell carcinoma
  Squamous cell carcinoma
  Adenocarcinoma

75. What is the type of change seen in patients with chronic alcoholism in the salivary gland?
    a. Hypoplasia
    b. Hyperplasia
    c. Fatty-tissue changes
    d. Higher glucose level

76. Dry mouth in a diabetic patient may be due to:
    a. Adiposis of the salivary gland
    b. Atrophy of the salivary gland
    c. Polyuria and poor hydration
    d. Fatty degeneration of the salivary gland

77. A possible reason suggested for salivary dysfunction in a diabetic patient may be:
    a. Adiposis of the salivary gland
    b. Atrophy of the salivary gland
    c. Fatty degeneration of the salivary gland
    d. Autonomic nervous system dysfunction

Ans. 75. c 76. c 77. d

78. One of the features associated with anorexia nervosa (bulimia) may be:
    a. Salivary gland enlargement and dysfunction
    b. Oral ulcerations
    c. Oral candidiasis
    d. Geographic tongue

79. Parotid salivary gland hypertrophy is best managed with:
    a. Mild radiation
    b. Sialogogues
    c. Superficial parotidectomy
    d. Complete excision of the gland

80. Salivary gland enlargement in alcoholic patients may be due to:
    a. Necrosis of the gland
    b. Fatty-tissue changes
    c. Toxic effects of alcohol on the gland tissue
    d. Malignant transformation

81. One of the commonest side-effects associated with the use of anticholinergics is:
    a. Xerostomia
    b. Lichenoid drug reaction
    c. Hepatotoxicity
    d. Sevens-Johnson syndrome

82. Benign lymphoepithelial lesion may be caused by all the following factors except:
    a. Autoimmune
    b. Viral
    c. Genetic
    d. Bacterial

83. Salivary gland enlargement may be caused by all except:
    a. Lymphoma
    b. Sarcoidosis
    c. Leukemia
    d. Sjögren's syndrome

84. The detection of monoclonal lymphocytic infiltrate is suggestive of:
    a. Low-grade lymphoma
    b. Megaloblastic anemia
    c. Pernicious anemia
    d. Addison's disease

Ans. 78. a 79. c 80. b 81. a 82. d 83. c 84. a

85. Among the following, which is not a feature of Sjögren's syndrome?
    a. Oral and ocular dryness
    b. Lymphocytic infiltration
    c. Destruction of the exocrine glands
    d. Metaplastic changes in the salivary gland

86. Among the following, which is not a feature of Sjögren's syndrome?
    a. Arthralgia
    b. Carditis
    c. Myalgia
    d. Rashes

87. Among the following statements about Sjögren's syndrome, which is incorrect?
    a. It usually affects post-menopausal women
    b. Female to male ratio is 9:1
    c. Classified as primary, secondary and tertiary
    d. Lacrimal and salivary gland dysfunction

88. What are the criteria to diagnose Sjögren's syndrome?

    There are no objective criteria to diagnose Sjögren's syndrome. However the following features may be suggestive of Sjögren's syndrome.
    - Decreased salivary gland function
    - Decreased lacrimal gland function
    - Positive autoimmune serologies
    - Minor salivary gland biopsy specimen demonstrating focal mononuclear cell infiltration in a periductal pattern

89. Minor salivary gland biopsy specimen demonstrating focal mononuclear cell infiltration in a periductal pattern is a feature of:
    a. Necrotizing sialometaplasia
    b. Discoid lupus erythematosus
    c. Sjögren's syndrome
    d. Mucocele

90. What is the grading system for quantifying the salivary histologic changes seen in the minor salivary glands in Sjögren's syndrome?
    - The numbers of infiltrating mononuclear cells are determined, with an aggregate of 50 or more cells being termed a focus
    - The total number of foci and the surface area of the specimen are measured

---

Ans. 85. d 86. b 87. c 89. c

- The number of foci per 4 mm^2 is calculated. This is the focus score. The range is from 0 to 12, with 12 denoting confluent infiltrates. A focus score of 1 is considered to be positive for Sjögren's syndrome .

91. Among the following drugs, which is not used in the trial of treating Sjögren's syndrome?
    a. Dehydroepiandrosterone (DHEA)
    b. Sex hormones
    c. Bleomycin
    d. Interferon-alpha

92. Incidence of which disease has been found to occur along with Sjögren's syndrome?
    a. Malignant lymphoma
    b. Squamous cell carcinoma
    c. AIDS
    d. Stevens-Johnson syndrome

93. Among the following statements about sarcoidosis, which is incorrect?
    a. Etiology is bacterial infection
    b. Onset primarily occurs in the 3rd and 4th decades
    c. Women are affected more than men
    d. African Americans are affected more than the Caucasians

94. Uveoparotid fever is a form of:
    a. Viral fever
    b. Bone marrow suppression
    c. Sarcoidosis
    d. Necrosis of salivary gland

95. Among the following, which is not a feature of uveoparotid fever?
    a. Inflammation of the uveal tract of the eye
    b. Stomatitis
    c. Parotid swelling
    d. Facial palsy

96. Serum evaluation indicating serum angiotensin I- converting enzyme concentration is indicative of:
    a. Sarcoidosis
    b. Sjögren's syndrome
    c. Tuberculosis
    d. AIDS

Ans. 91. c 92. a 93. a 94. c 95. b 96. a

97. Among the following, which is not a drug used in the management of acute phases of sarcoidosis?
    a. Corticosteroids
    b. Anticholinergics
    c. Chloroquine
    d. Immunosuppressive medications

98. The infection that patients with xerostomia can experience is:
    a. Bacterial sialadenitis
    b. Candidiasis
    c. HSV infection
    d. Parasitic infection

99. Among the following which is not used as a secretogogue for salivary stimulation?
    a. Bromhexine
    b. Anetholetrithione
    c. Pilocarpine hydrochloride
    d. Clevulinic acid

100. Bromhexine is:
    a. Immunomodulator
    b. Mucolytic agent
    c. Antiinflammatory
    d. Antibiotic

Ans. 97. b 98. b 99. d 100. b

SECTION VI

1. Anetholetrithione is:
   a. Immunomodulator
   b. Mucolytic agent
   c. Antiinflammatory drug
   d. Antipyretic
2. Pilocarpine hydrochloride is:
   a. Parasympathomimetic
   b. Antiinflammatory
   c. Antibiotic
   d. Cholinergic anagonist
3. The best tolerated dose of pilocarpine three or four times daily in the treatment of xerostomia is:
   a. 0.5 to 0.75 mg
   b. 5.0 to 7.5 mg
   c. 50 to 75 mg
   d. 500 to 750 mg
4. Among the following, which is not a contraindication for pilocarpine?
   a. Pulmonary disease
   b. Asthma
   c. Cardiovascular disease
   d. Nephrotic syndrome
5. One of the features associated with administration of pilocarpine is:
   a. Xerostomia
   b. Sialorrhea
   d. Salivary gland atresia
   d. Salivary gland hypertrophy
6. Injection of botulinum toxin into the glands of patients with neurologic disease can result in:
   a. Decreased saliva flow
   b. Increased saliva flow
   c. Necrosis of salivary gland
   d. Hyperplasia of the salivary gland

Ans. 1. b 2. a 3. b 4. d 5. b 6. a

7. Majority of salivary gland tumours arise from:
   a. Minor salivary glands
   b. Parotid salivary gland
   c. Submandibular salivary gland
   d. Sublingual salivary gland

8. The most common salivary gland tumour is:
   a. Monomorphic adenoma
   b. Pleomorohic adenoma
   c. Oncocytoma
   d. Papillary cystadenoma lymphomatosum

9. Intraorally, the most favourable location of pleomorphic adenoma is:
   a. Palate
   b. Buccal mucosa
   c. Floor of the mouth
   d. Parotid papilla

10. The epithelial cells making up a trabecular pattern that is contained within a stroma which may be chondroid, myxoid, osteoid or fibroid is a feature of:
    a. Pleomorphic adenoma
    b. Monomorphic adenoma
    c. Oncocytoma
    d. Papillary cystadenoma lymphomatosum

11. Microscopic projections of tumour outside of the capsule is a feature of:
    a. Pleomorphic adenoma
    b. Monomorphic adenoma
    c. Oncocytoma
    d. Papillary cystadenoma lymphomatosum

12. Histologically, the stroma in pleomorphic adenoma may be the following except:
    a. Chondroid
    b. Myxoid
    c. Fibroid
    d. Collagenoid

13. Warthin's tumour refers to:
    a. Pleomorphic adenoma
    b. Monomorphic adenoma
    c. Papillary cystadenoma lymphomatosum
    d. Oncocytoma

Ans. 7. b 8. b 9. a 10. a 11. a 12. d 13. c

14. The most favoured site (in the parotid salivary gland) of occurrence of Warthin's tumour is:
    a. Superficial lobe
    b. Deep lobe
    c. Posterior lobe
    d. Inferior pole
15. Histologically, presence of papillary projections lined with eosinophilic cells that project into cystic spaces may be a feature of:
    a. Pleomorphic adenoma
    b. Monomorphic adenoma
    c. Warthin's tumour
    d. Oncocytoma
16. Among the following, which is the rarest tumour affecting the salivary glands?
    a. Pleomorphic adenoma
    b. Monomorphic adenoma
    c. Warthin's tumour
    d. Oncocytoma
17. Oncocytoma affects which salivary gland?
    a. Parotd
    b. Submandibular
    c. Sublingual
    d. Accessory
18. Among the following statements about oncocytoma, which is wrong?
    a. It contains oncocytes
    b. It is the most common salivary gland neoplasm
    c. It affects the parotid gland
    d. Sixth decade is the most common time of presentation
19. Oncocytomas are best treated by:
    a. Radiotherapy
    b. Radical excision
    c. Chemotherapy
    d. Superficial parotidectomy
20. Histologically, presence of granular eosinophilic cells is a feature of which salivary gland tumour?
    a. Oncocytoma
    b. Pleomorphic adenoma
    c. Monomorphic adenoma
    d. Papillary cystadenoma lymphomatosum

Ans. 14. d 15. c 16. d 17. a 18. b 19. d 20. a

21. Among the following statements about basal cell adenomas, which is incorrect?
    a. They are slow growing and painless masses
    b. There is a high female predilection
    c. Most of the cases are reported in the parotid gland
    d. Upper lip is the common site of presentation if minor salivary glands are involved

22. Among the following, which is not a type of basal cell adenoma?
    a. Solid
    b. Trabecular-tubular
    c. Membranous
    d. Papillary

23. Histologically, prsence of islands or sheets of basaloid cells with normal-sized nuclei which are basophilic with minimal cytoplasmic material may be a feature of:
    a. Squamous cell carcinoma
    b. Osteogenic sarcoma
    c. Basal cell adenoma
    d. Oral submucous fibrosis

24. Myoepitheliomas predominantly occur in which salivary gland?
    a. Parotid
    b. Submandibular
    c. Sublingual
    d. Accessory

25. Long strands of basaloid tissue, usually arranged in a double row with the supporting which is loose, fibrillar and highly vascular is a feature of:
    a. Canalicular adenoma
    b. Basal cell adenoma
    c. Papillary cystadenoma lymphomatosum
    d. Adenocarcinoma

26. The common site of occurrence of intraoral myoepithelioma is:
    a. Tongue
    b. Palate
    c. Biccal mucosa
    d. Tonsillar region

27. Which tumour is demonstrated by immunohistochemical staining for actin?
    a. Myoepithelioma
    b. Oncocytoma
    c. Basal cell adenoma
    d. Papillary cysadenoma lymphomatosum

Ans. 21. b 22. d 23. c 24. a 25. a 26. b 27. a

28. Ductal papillomas mainly affect which salivary gland?
    a. Parotid
    b. Submandibular
    c. Sublingual
    d. Minor

29. Among the following, which is not a type of ductal papilloma?
    a. Intraductal
    b. Inverted ductal
    c. Superficial ductal
    d. Sialadenoma papilliferum

30. The most common malignant salivary gland tumour is:
    a. Mucoepidermoid carcinoma
    b. Adenoid cystic carcinoma
    c. Acinic cell carcinoma
    d. Squamous cell carcinoma

31. Perineural invasion is a feature of which salivary gland tumour?
    a. Adenoid cystic carcinoma
    b. Mucoepidermoid carcinoma
    c. Acinic cell carcinoma
    d. Squamous cell carcinoma

32. Which salivary gland tumour is capable of spreading through the nerve sheaths?
    a. Adenoid cystic carcinoma
    b. Mucoepidermoid carcinoma
    c. Acinic cell carcinoma
    d. Squamous cell carcinoma

33. What is carcinoma ex pleomorphic adenoma?
    a. Carcinoma that exhibits the features of pleomorphic adenoma also
    b. Carcinoma that arises within a pre-existing pleomorphic adenoma
    c. Pleomorphic adenoma mimicking carcinoma
    d. Difficult lesion to differentiate between carcinoma and pleomorphic adenoma

34. What is the origin of carcinoma ex pleomorphic adenoma?
    a. Epithelial
    b. Mesenchymal
    c. Nerve cell
    d. Myoepithelial

Ans. 28. d 29. c 30. a 31. a 32. a 33. b 34. a

35. Any tumours arising from salivary duct epithelium are, by definition:
   a. Squamous cell carcinoma
   b. Adenocarcinoma
   c. Carcinoma-in-situ
   d. Oncocytoma

36. A tumour which can affect patients with autoimmune disease is:
   a. Squamous cell carcinoma
   b. Metastatic carcinoma
   c. Non-Hodgkin's lymphoma
   d. Malignant melanoma

37. Most of the tumours involving the parotid salivary gland are treated by:
   a. Surgical excision
   b. Superficial parotidectomy
   c. Laser therapy
   d. Radiotherapy

38. A complication of parotidectomy is:
   a. Sinus tract formation
   b. Necrosis of the facial muscles
   c. Frey's syndrome
   d. Trigeminal neuralgia

39. Gustatory sweating is seen in case of:
   a. Frey's syndrome
   b. Weech's syndrome
   c. Beckwith's hypoglycemic syndrome
   d. Ehlers-Danlos syndrome

40. Area of gustatory sweating can be demonstrated by:
   a. Injecting contrast
   b. Fluoroscopy
   c. Minor's starch iodine test
   d. Analyzing the taste perception

41. Among the following, which may not be a complication associated with parotidectomy?
   a. Permanent or total facial nerve paralysis
   b. Alteration of taste perception
   c. Salivary fistula or sialocele
   d. Temporary nerve palsies

Ans. 35. b 36. c 37. b 38. c 39. a 40. c 41. b

42. Sialocele formation occurs as a result of:
    a. Xerostomia
    b. Infection of the sallivary gland
    c. Due to the damage of the capsule and resltant pooling of saliva
    d. Air entrapment within the salivary gland duct

43. What are the cardinal symptoms of temporomandibular disorders (TMDs)?

    There are certain basic clinical features associated with temporomandibular disorders. These are the following:
    - Facial pain in the region of the temporomandibular joint (TMJ)
    - Pain involving the masticatory muscles
    - Limitation or deviation of the mandible during mandibular range of movements
    - Joint sounds during jaw movement and function

44. In the TMJ, the bony components are enclosed and connected by:
    a. Loose areolar tissue
    b. Ligaments
    c. Tendon
    d. Fibrous capsule

45. In the TMJ, the condyle occupies the fossa in the:
    a. Temporal bone
    b. Sphenoid bone
    c. Parietal bone
    d. Occipital bone

46. At what age does the glenoid fossa and the articular eminence develop?
    a. 6th week of IU life
    b. 3rd week after birth
    c. 6 years of age
    d. 9 month of age

47. In the TMJ, the joint cavity is filled with:
    a. Serum
    b. Synovial fluid
    c. Fat
    d. Transudate

48. Synovial tissue is basically:
    a. Adipose tissue
    b. Nerve tissue
    c. Muscle tissue
    d. Vascular connective tissue

Ans. 42. c 44. d 45. a 46. c 47. b 48. d

49. Synovial fluid is basically:
    a. Inflammatory edema
    b. Serum
    c. Filtrate of plasma
    d. Interstitial body fluid

50. The main constituent of synovial fluid is:
    a. Protein
    b. Aminoacid
    c. Hyaluronic acid
    d. Lipid

51. The lining of TMJ is by:
    a. Fibrocartilage
    b. Hyaline cartilage
    c. Loose areolar tissue
    d. Tendon

52. Among the following, which is the most important property of fibrocartilage?
    a. Highly elastic
    b. Less distensible
    c. Ability to deform
    d. Ability to absorb stress

53. Among the following, which is not present in the articular disk?
    a. Collagen fibres
    b. Proteoglycans
    c. Elastic fibres
    d. Osteoid material

54. The collagen fibres of the articular disk in the center are oriented in which direction to its transverse axis?
    a. Parallel
    b. Vertical
    c. Perpendicular
    d. Circular

55. The compressive stiffness of the articular cartilage is influenzed by:
    a. Calcification
    b. Presence of muscle fibres
    c. Cartilage-like proteoglycans
    d. Osteoblasts

56. The ligaments attached to the medial and lateral poles of the condyle permit which type of movement?
    a. Rotational movement
    b. Translational movement
    c. Vertical movement
    d. Transverse movement

Ans. 49. c 50. c 51. a 52. b 53. d 54. c 55. c 56. a

57. Among the following statements about the articular disk, which is false?

   a. The articular disk is composed of collagenous and fibrous tissue
   b. The disc is avascular and has little sensory nerve penetration
   c. The disk is attached to the medial and lateral poles of the condyle by ligaments
   d. The disk is thickest in the center and and thins to form anterior and posterior bands at the ends

58. The upper and lower compartments of the joint:

   a. Always communicate
   b. Normally do not communicate
   c. Communicate during mouth opening
   d. Communicate during closing

59. The floor of the superior compartment of the TMJ is by:

   a. Superior surface of the disc
   b. Mandibular fossa
   c. Condylar head
   d. Petrotympanic fissure

60. The roof of the inferior compartment is made up of ;

   a. Superior surface of the disc
   b. Mandibular fossa
   c. Inferior surface of the disc
   d. Petrotympanic fissure

61. Fibres of the posterior one-third of the temporalis muscle and and deep masseter muscle may attach at which part of the disk in theTMJ?

   a. Anterolateral
   b. Posterolateral
   c. Superolateral
   d. Inferolateral

62. What is present in the space behind the disk and condyle?

   a. Nerve fibres
   b. Dense fibrocartilage
   c. Dense collagen fibres
   d. Mass of soft tissue

Ans. 57. d 58. b 59. a 60. c 61. a 62. d

63. What is the posterior attachment of the articular disk?
    a. A soft tissue mass behind the disk and the condyle
    b. Nerve fibres
    c. Fibrocartilage
    d. Dense collagen fibres

64. The main ligament of the TMJ is:
    a. Capsular ligament
    b. Stylomandibular ligament
    c. Sphenomandibular ligament
    d. Retrodiscal tissue

65. Among the following, which is not a muscle of mastication?
    a. Masseter
    b. Temporalis
    c. Myelohyoid
    d. Medial and lateral pterygoid

66. Contraction of which masticatory muscle helps in the movement of condylar head towards the anterior slope of the mandibular fossa?
    a. Masseter
    b. Temporalis
    c. Medial pterygoid
    d. Lateral pterygoid

67. Among the following, which is not an accessory muscle of mastication?
    a. Mylohyoid
    b. Geniohyoid
    c. Digastric
    d. Lateral pterygoid

68. Which mandibular function is performed by the mylohyoid and geniohyoid muscles?
    a. Protrusion
    b. Depression
    c. Elevation
    d. Lateral movement

69. The main arterial supply of the TMJ is by:
    a. Facial artery
    b. External carotid artery
    c. Occipital artery
    d. There is no arterial supply to TMJ as it is avascular

Ans. 63. a 64. b 65. c 66. a 67. d 68. b 69. b

70. Among the following cranial nerves, which does not innervate the TMJ?

a. IV
b. V
c. IX
d. VII

71. Sensory innervation of the TMJ is by:

a. Deep temporal nerve
b. Auriculotemporal nerve
c. Masseteric nerve
d. Buccal nerve

72. What position is occupied by the condyle with respect to the mandibular fossa during rest position?

a. Superior aspect
b. Inferior aspect
c. Middle aspect
d. Anterior aspect

73. Excessive jaw opening is governed by all the following except:

a. Temporomandibular ligament
b. Stylomandibular ligament
c. Articular eminence
d. Dentition

74. The greatest functional load falls on which area of the fibrocartilage?

a. Posterior slope of the articular eminence and on the anterior slope of the condylar head
b. Anterior slope of the articular eminence and the anterior slope of the condylar head
c. Posterior slope of the articular eminence and on the posterior slope of the condylar head
d. Anterior slope of the articular eminence and the posterior slope of the condylar head

75. Anterior disk displacement may be associated with dysfunction of which muscle?

a. Temporalis
b. Masseter
c. Medial pterygoid
d. Lateral pterygoid

Ans. 70. a 71. b 72. c 73. d 74. a 75. d

76. The site of TMJ injections should be:
   a. Anterior to the tragus
   b. Posterior to the tragus
   c. Superior to the tragus
   d. Inferior to the tragus

77. Fibres of which muscle is intimately associated to the lateral wall of the joint capsule?
   a. Temporalis
   b. Masseter
   c. Medial pterygoid
   d. Lateral pterygoid

78. Which are the most common etiological factors for temporomandibular disorders (TMD)?

   The exact etiological factors responsible for TMD are not known. But the commonest causes are the following:
   - Occlusal disharmony
   - Psychological stress
   - Parafunctional habits such as bruxism, tooth clenching, lip biting and cheek biting
   - Acute trauma from blows or impact
   - Trauma from hyperextension
   - Instability of maxillomandibular relationships
   - Laxity of the joint
   - Comorbidity of other rheumatic or musculoskeletal disorders
   - Poor general health and an unhealthy lifestyle

79. Which is the most accessible part for palpation of the condyle?
   a. Medial
   b. Lateral
   c. Anterior
   d. Posterior

80. Which are the various diagnostic modalities available for TMJ evaluation?

   There are various diagnostic modalities available for the evaluation of TMJ. These are:
   - Conventional radiographs (TMJ views)
   - Tomography
   - Arthrography
   - Computerized tomography (CT0
   - Magnetic resonance imaging (MRI)
   - Single-photon emission computed tomography
   - Radioisotope scanning

Ans. 76. a 77. b 79. b 80.

81. What is the advantage of using MRI in the evaluation of TMJ?
    a. It helps in identifying any pathology involving the bony elements
    b. It helps in the detection of accumulated inflammatory edema
    c. It helps to assess the disk position
    d. It helps in monitoring the functional activity of the TMJ

82. Osteodegenerative changes involving the TMJ are best evaluated by:
    a. Transcranial view
    b. Magnetic resonance imaging
    c. Arthrography
    d. Tomography and CT

83. Metabolic bone activity of the TMJ is best evaluated by:
    a. Bone scanning
    b. MRI
    c. Tomography and CT scan
    d. Arthrography

84. Which are the methods available in physiotherapy for the management of temporomandibular disorders?

    The following are the various methods available in the physiotherapy for the management of TMD:
    - Ultrasound
    - Laser therapy
    - Transcutaneous electrical nerve stimulation (TENS)
    - Jaw exercises
    - Mobilization techniques

85. Degenerative joint disease mainly affects:
    a. Articular disk
    b. Articular cartilage and subchondral bone
    c. Masticatory muscles
    d. Accessory muscles of mastication

86. Multiple cartilaginous nodules of the synovial membrane breaking off, resulting in free-floating loose calcified bodies in the joint is a condition called:
    a. Degenerative joint disease
    b. Rheumatoid arthritis
    c. Psoriatic arthritis
    d. Chondrometaplasia

Ans. 81. c 82. d 83. a 85. b 86. d

87. A severe case of psoriatic arthritis is managed with:
    a. Gold salts
    b. Methotrexate
    c. NSAIDs
    d. Injection of steroids into the joint

88. The main primary organism which is capable of causing septic arthritis involving the TMJ is:
    a. Staphylococci
    b. Streptococci
    c. Pneumococci
    d. Gonococi

89. Long-term elevation of serum urate levels can result in:
    a. Rheumatoid arthritis
    b. Degenerative joint disease
    c. Gout
    d. Psoriatic arthritis

90. Crystal deposition adjacent to the joint is seen in:
    a. Rheumatoid arthritis
    b. Gout
    c. Psoriatic arthritis
    d. Ankylosis

91. Deposition of crystals such as calcium pyrophosphate dihydrate (CPPD) or calcium hydroxyapatite in the joint is called:
    a. Pseudogout
    b. Dystrophic calcification
    c. Rheumatoid arthritis
    d. Psoriatic arthritis

92. A case of pseudogout involving the TMJ is managed with:
    a. NSAIDs
    b. Antibiotics
    c. Methotrexate
    d. Colchicine

93. The most reliable method to diagnose gout involving the TMJ is by:
    a. MRI
    b. Arthrography
    c. Aspiration and microscopic evaluation of synovial fluid
    d. TMJ arthropanoromography

Ans. 87. b 88. d 89. c 90. b 91. a 92. d 93. c

94. Still's disease refers to:
    a. Childhood rheumatoid arthritis
    b. Occurrence of severe stomatitis
    c. Occurrence of intraoral and extraoral lichen planus
    d. Developmental disturbance and mental retardation

95. Which is the dominant cranial nerve that relays sensory impulses from the orofacial region to the central nervous system (CNS)?
    a. II
    b. III
    c. IV
    d. V

96. Visual analog scale is used for:
    a. Detecting mouth opening
    b. To identify mandibular deviation
    c. To measure pain intensity
    d. To determine colour blindness

97. Allodynia refers to:
    a. Facial pain and facial paralysis
    b. Pain due to a stimulus that does not normally provoke pain
    c. Pain involving the tongue
    d. Burning mouth syndrome

98. Pressure algometers are used for:
    a. Determining blood pressure
    b. Standardizing muscle palpation
    c. Performing capillary fragility test
    d. For pulp vitality test

99. Which are the systemic diseases associated with headache and orofacial pain?

    The following are the various systemic diseases associated with headache and orofacial pain:
    - Paget's disease
    - Metastatic disease
    - Hyperthyroidism
    - Multiple myeloma
    - Hyperparathyroidism
    - Vitamin B deficiencies
    - Systemic lupus erythematosus (SLE)
    - Vincristine therapy for cancer
    - Folic acid and iron deficiency anemia

Ans. 94. a 95. d 96. c 97. b 98. b

100. Which are the conditions which may be confused with toothache?

The following are the conditions which may be cofused with toothache:

- Trigeminal neuralgia
- Trigeminal neuropathy (due to trauma or tumour invasion of nerve)
- Atypical facial pain
- Atypical odontalgia
- Cluster headache
- Acute and chronic maxillary sinusitis
- Myofascial pain of masticatory muscles

Ans.

SECTION VII

1. The most frequent tumour associated with the etiology of trigeminal neuralgia is:
   a. Squamous cell carcinoma
   b. Meningioma
   c. Paget's disease
   d. Fibrous dysplasia
2. What is the concept about the cause for pressure of the trigeminal nerve in case of trigeminal neuralgia?
   a. Atherosclerotic blood vessel
   b. Inelastic blood vessel
   c. Embolism
   d. Squamous cell carcinoma of maxillary sinus
3. What are "trigger zones"?
   a. Areas in the mouth where cancer originates
   b. Areas on the skin and mucosa, when touched pain impulse is generated
   c. Areas likely to be infected by HIV virus
   d. Areas of malignant transformation in premalignant lesions
4. Which are the best drugs for managing trigeminal neuralgia?
   a. Analgesics
   b. Anticonvulsants
   c. Antimetabolites
   d. Antihypertensives
5. Which is a newer anticonvulsant that is found to be effective in the treatment of trigeminal neuralgia?
   a. Carbamazepine
   b. Baclofen
   c. Gabapentin
   d. Dilantin
6. Anticonvulsants such as carbamazepine are administered in:
   a. Tapering dosage
   b. Incereasing dosage
   c. Aggressive dosage
   d. Intermittent dosage

Ans. 1. b 2. a 3. b 4. b 5. c 6. b

7. Among the following areas, which may not be a trigger zone for glossopharyngeal neuralgia?
   a. Pharynx
   b. Posterior tongue
   c. Ear
   d. Occiput
8. The neuralgia more likely to cause syncope and arrhythmia due to vagal stimulation is:
   a. Trigeminal neuralgia
   b. Glossopharyngeal neuralgia
   c. Atypical facial fain
   d. Geniculate neuralgia
9. Elimination of glossopharyngeal nerve pain is achieved by:
   a. Inferior alveolar nerve block
   b. Application of topical anesthetic to pharyngeal mucosa
   c. Stimulating vagus nerve
   d. Injection of anesthetic into the oropharynx
10. The most common causes for glossopharyngeal neuralgia are:
    a. Bacterial and viral infections
    b. Exposure to wind and cold breeze
    c. Intracranial or extracranial tumours
    d. Severe pharyngitis and tonsillitis
11. Which drug can be used in the treatment of glosssopharyngeal neuralgia?
    a. Baclofen
    b. Proxyvon
    c. NSAIDs
    d. Alcohol (as injection)
12. Radifrequency thermocoagulation is a procedure for:
    a. Measurement of radiation exposure
    b. Treatment of trigeminal nuralgia
    c. Treatment of leukoplakia
    d. Determination of X-ray film sensitivity
13. Nervus intermedius or geniculate neuralgia affects which cranial nerve?
    a. IV
    b. V
    c. VI
    d. VII
14. Geniculate neuralgia affects which sensory area?
    a. Pharyngeal mucosa and tongue
    b. External surface of the face
    c. External auditory canal and soft palate
    d. Forehead

Ans. 7. d 8. b 9. b 10. c 11. a 12. b 13. d 14. c

15. Herpes zoster of geniculate ganglion and nervus intermedius causes:
    a. Trigeminal neuralgia
    b. Ramsay Hunt syndrome
    c. Cerebellopontine angle tumour
    d. Occipital neuralgia
16. Which treatment modality may be beneficial in a patient with Ramsay Hunt syndrome?
    a. Injection of sclerosing solutions
    b. High-dose steroids
    c. Antibiotics
    d. Aspirin
17. Among the following which is not a cause for occipital neuralgia?
    a. Trauma
    b. Infections
    c. Aneurysms
    d. Radiation
18. A tender spot during palpation below superior nuchal line is suggestive of:
    a. Trigeminal neuralgia
    b. Occipital neuralgia
    c. Glossopharyngeal neuralgia
    d. Geniculate neuralgia
19. The individuals more likely to be affected by post-herpetic neuralgia are:
    a. Post-menopausal women
    b. Elderly
    c. Infants
    d. Young adults
20. Demyelination, wallerian degeneration and scoliosis are features of:
    a. Varicella-zoster infection
    b. Post-herpetic neuralgia
    c. Injuries due to burn
    d. Scleroderma
21. Shingles refers to:
    a. HIV infection
    b. Herpes zoster
    c. Chicken pox
    d. Mumps

Ans. 15. b 16. b 17. d 18. b 19. b 20. a 21. b

22. Post herpetic neuralgia is best managed with:
    a. Acyclovir
    b. Topical application of lidocaine
    c. Carbamazepine
    d. Baclofen

23. Axonotmesis refers to:
    a. Serious nerve damage
    b. Post herpetic neuralgia
    c. Stimulation of trigger zones causing pain in trigeminal neuralgia
    d. Involvement of nerve by viruses

24. Neurapraxia refers to:
    a. Post herpetic neuralgia
    b. Stimulation of trigger zones causing pain in trigeminal neuralgia
    c. Involvement of nerve by viruses
    d. Minor nerve damage

25. Among the following statements about cranial arteritis, which is wrong?
    a. It is caused by immune abnormalities
    b. Affects cytokines and B lymphocytes
    c. Causes inflammatory infiltrates in the walls of arteries
    d. There is formation of multinucleated giant cells

26. A serious complication of ischemia of the eye in untreated patients is characteristic of:
    a. Maxillary sinusitis
    b. Osteomyelitis
    c. Temporal arteritis
    d. Paget's disease

27. Laboratory studies revealing abnormal C-reactive protein may be a feature of:
    a. Lichen planus   b. Temporal arteritis
    c. Rheumatoid arthritis
    d. Diabetes mellitus

28. Chronic pounding head or orofacial pain and an elevated ESR in a patient over 50 years of age should be considered as:
    a. Hypertension   b. Diabetes mellitus
    c. Renal disease   d. Temporal arteritis

Ans. 22. b 23. a 24. d 25. b 26. c 27. b 28. d

29. The drug usually employed in the treatment of temporal arteritis is:
    a. Penicillin
    b. Prednisone
    c. Calcium channel blockers
    d. Aspirin

30. Which drug is used in association with corticosteroids in the management of temporal arteritis?
    a. Aspirin
    b. Calcium channel blocker
    c. Cyclophosphamide
    d. Penicillin

31. Episodes of severe unilateral head pain occurring chiefly around the eye and accompanied by a number of autonomic signs is characteristic of:
    a. Trigeminal neuralgia
    b. Cluster headache
    c. Atypical facial pain
    d. Epilepsy

32. An acute attack of cluster headache can be aborted by:
    a. Breathing oxygen
    b. Injecting adrenaline
    c. Sublingual nitroglycerine
    d. Morphine

33. Among the following, which is not a form of migraine?
    a. Atypical
    b. Classic
    c. Basilar
    d. Facial

34. Carotidynia is also called as:
    a. Facial migraine
    b. Trigeminal neuralgia
    c. Temporal arteritis
    d. Atypical facial pain

35. Which drug is used to manage difficult cases of migraine?
    a. Ergotamine
    b. Propranolol
    c. Verapamil
    d. Phenelzine

Ans. 29. b 30. c 31. b 32. a 33. a 34. a 35. d

36. A possible side-effect of using long-term glucocorticosteroid inhalers may be:

    a. Nasopharyngeal necrosis
    b. Candidiasis
    c. Ulcerations
    d. Allergic response

37. Majority of upper respiratory infections in adults are caused by which virus?

    a. Rhinovirus
    b. Epstein Barr
    c. HSV
    d. Paramyxovirus

38. Which are the viruses associated with causing upper respiratory tract infections?

    The following are the viruses associated with causing upper respiratory tract infections:

    - Rhinoviruses
    - Coronavirus
    - Influenza virus
    - Parainfluenza virus
    - Adenovirus
    - Enterovirus
    - Coxsackievirus
    - Respiratory syncytial virus

39. The end result of sensitization in allergic response is production of which specific immunoblobulin?

    a. A
    b. D
    c. E
    d. M

40. Otitis media refers to:

    a. Inflammation of middle-ear space and tissues
    b. Inflammation of middle carnial fossa
    c. Inflammation of midline of the face
    d. Cavernous sinus thrombosis

41. Pansinusitis refers to:

    a. Simultaneous inflammatory involvement of all the sinuses
    b. Sinus inflammation seen among pan chewers
    c. Inflammatory involvement of maxillary and frontal sinuses
    d. A complication associated with maxillary sinusitis characterized by severe necrosis

---

Ans. 36. b 37. a 39. c 40. a 41. a

42. The best diagnostic modality in the evaluation of osteomeatal complex disease is:
    a. Plain-film sinus radiography
    b. CT
    c. MRI
    d. Bone scan

43. Pott's puffy tumour refers to:
    a. Frontal sinusitis extending through the anterior wall
    b. Chronic osteomyelitis involving the maxillary sinus
    c. Oral manifestation of Cushing's syndrome
    d. Inability to puff the mouth in case of Bell's palsy

44. The most common bacterial cause for tonsillopharyngitis is:
    a. Gonococcus
    b. Staphylococcus
    c. Beta-hemolytic Streptococcus
    d. Streptococcus pyogenes

45. Exudative tonsillopharyngitis is a feature of:
    a. Beta-hemolytic streptococcus infection
    b. Herpangina
    c. Infectious mononucleosis
    d. Agranulocytosis

46. Koplik's spots are characteristic of:
    a. Measles
    b. Infectious mononucleosis
    c. Rubella
    d. Rubeola

47. Koplik's spots are predominantly seen in:
    a. Palate
    b. Tonsillar region
    c. Tongue and mucobuccal fold
    d. Buccal mucosa and lower lip

48. Small white lesions with erythematous bases seen on the buccal mucosa and inner aspect of the lower lip are called:
    a. Stomatitis medicamentosa
    b. Koplik's spots
    c. Fordyce granules
    d. Heck's disease

Ans. 42. b 43. a 44. c 45. a 46. a 47. d 48. b

49. Koplik's spots are seen in:
   a. Prodromal phase of measles infection
   b. Early stage of measles infection
   c. Advanced case of measles infection
   d. Complication of measles infection

50. Beefy red uvula, cervical adenitis and oral petechiae are characteristic of:
   a. Infectious mononucleosis
   b. Streptococcal pharyngitis
   c. Herpangina
   d. Agranulocytosis

51. The commonest cause for bronchitis is:
   a. Virus b. Bacteria
   c. Fungi d. Parasites

52. What is the dental significance of bronchitis?

The drug of choice in the management of bronchitis as amoxicillin. As occurrence of antibiotic resistance is likely to develop rapidly which can even last for 10 to 14 days, a concomitant odontogenic infection may have to be treated with another type of antibiotic such as clindamycin or cephalosporin.

53. In the pathophysiology of pneumonia, the initial involvement is:
   a. Upper respiratory tract
   b. Larynx
   c. Bronchi
   d. Alveoli

54. In the healing phase of bacterial pneumonia, deposition of —— ensues as the infection is controlled:
   a. Polymorphonuclear leukocytes
   b. Macrophages
   c. Fibrin
   d. Epithelium

55. Elevated liver enzymes and proteinuria indicate renal and hepatic involvement in case of:
   a. Bronchitis b. Pneumonia
   c. Legionnaire's disease d. Tuberculosis

Ans. 49. b 50. b 51. a 53. d 54. c 55. c

56. Radiographically a pattern of globar consolidation and air bronchograms are seen most predominantly in case of:
    a. Pneumococcal pneumonia
    b. Bronchitis
    c. Bronchiectasis
    d. Pulmonary tuberculosis

57. Cold agglutinins refer to:
    a. Antibodies produced against allergens
    b. Antibodies produced against Mycoplasma infection
    c. Antibodies produced against virus
    d. Antibodies produced against systemic infection

58. Which is the antibiotic of choice in the management of pneumonia caused by *Legionella* or *Mucoplasma*?
    a. Amoxicillin
    b. Ampicillin
    c. Cephalosporin
    d. Erythromycin

59. Among the following statements about bronchiolitis, which is incorrect?
    a. It affects elderly individuals
    b. It is characterized by inflammation of the lower respiratory tract
    c. Infectious trigger is usually respiratory syncytial virus (RSV)
    d. Occasionally it can cause bronchiolar spasm

60. On chest radiography, peribronchial cuffing, flattening of the diaphragms, hyperinflation and increased lung markings are characteristic of:
    a. Bronchitis
    b. Tuberculosis
    c. Pneumonia
    d. Bronchiolitis

61. Spirometry is the best tool available in the diagnosis and management of which disease?
    a. Asthma
    b. Bronchitis
    c. Pneumonia
    d. Bronchiolitis

62. Allergen immunotherapy is indicated in the treatment of which condition?
    a. Asthma
    b. Bronchitis
    c. Pneumonia
    d. Bronchiolitis

Ans. 56. a 57. b 58. d 59. a 60. d 61. a 62. a

63. What are the dental considerations of bronchial asthma?

The following are the dental considerations associated with bronchial asthma:

- Repeated use of corticosteroid inhalers can lead to oropharyngeal candidiasis
- Use of bronchodilators such as ipratropium bromide can cause xerostomia
- Acute asthmatic attack can be precipitated by stressful dental procedures. To avoid stress, sedation may be required
- Whenever patients with bronchial asthma report for dental treatment, they should bring their medication along
- Patients having bronchial asthma should not be given non-steroidal anti-inflammatory drugs (NSAIDs) such as aspirin, mefenemic acid, paracetamol or pentazocine, as these drugs can induce bronchospasm and thus precipitating an attack of bronchial asthma
- As patients with bronchial asthma are prone for hypoxia and hypercapnia, general anesthesia (GA) should be avoided in these patients

64. Cystic fibrosis is also called as:
   a. Bronchiectasis
   b. Chronic obstructive pulmonary disease (COPD)
   c. Mucoviscidosis
   d. Bronchiolitis

65. Cystic fibrosis affects:
   a. Fibroblasts
   b. Blood vessels
   c. Nerves
   d. Exocrine glands

66. Cystic fibrosis is caused by:
   a. Infection
   b. Immunologic causes
   c. Inflammatory process
   d. Inherited error of metabolism

67. Pancreatic insufficiency due to blockage of the pancreatic duct by mucus with malabsorption leading to bulky and foul-smelling stool are features of:
   a. Sprue
   b. Cystic fibrosis
   c. Bacillary dysentery
   d. Intestinal malabsorption

Ans. 64. c 65. d 66. d 67. b

68. Mantoux test is done for the diagnosis of:
    a. Hansen's disease
    b. Oral squamous cell carcinoma
    c. Sarcoidosis
    d. Tuberculosis

69. Chronic hypoxemia, pulmonary hypertension, right ventricular hypertrophy and cardiac failure are features of:
    a. Shock
    b. Pulmonary embolism
    c. Stroke
    d. COPD

70. Kveim test is indicated in:
    a. Bronchitis
    b. Sarcoidosis
    c. Hansen's disease
    d. Tuberculosis

71. What is Kveim test?

    Kveim test is a diagnostic test for sarcoidosis. This test is performed as follows:
    - Heat-sterilized suspension of human spleen or lymph node affected by sarcoidosis is injected subcutaneously
    - After 4 to 6 weeks, the injected area is biopsied and examined for epitheloid granulomas
    - The test gives positive test result in about 80% of cases

72. What is the treatment modality for sarcoidosis?
    a. Chemotherapy
    b. Radiotherapy
    c. Corticosteroids
    d. Antibiotics

73. Among the following, which is not a feature of Heerfordt's syndome?
    a. Salivary and lacrimal gland enlargement
    b. Fever
    c. Uveitis
    d. Blepharochalasis

74. An opening between the aorta and pulmonary artery is called:
    a. Ventricular septal defect
    b. Patent ductus arteriosus
    c. Atrial septal defect
    d. Coarctation of aorta

Ans. 68. d 69. d 70. b 72. c 73. d 74. b

75. Right ventricular hypertrophy, reversal of the shunt, cyanosis, right ventricular failure, endocardial thickening due to jet-like blood flow (jet lesion) are features of:
   a. Atrial septal defect
   b. Ventricular septal defect
   c. Patent ductus arteriosus
   d. Coarctation of aorta

76. The commonest cause for chronic obstructive pulmonary disease is:
   a. Bacterial infection
   b. Viral infection
   c. Smoking
   d. Enzyme deficiency

77. Functional impairment of enzymes that are required for respiratory metabolism is caused by:
   a. Hydrogen peroxide
   b. Hydrogen cyanide
   c. Nitrosomines
   d. Carbon monoxide

78. Measurement of arterial blood gases are helpful in the diagnosis of:
   a. Pulmonary embolism
   b. Bronchiectasis
   c. Bronchiolitis
   d. COPD

79. What are the risk factors of cardiovascular diseases?

   The following arc the risk factors of cardiovascular diseases:
   - Smoking
   - Dyslipidemia
   - Diabetes mellitus
   - Above 50 years of age
   - Male patients
   - Postmenopause
   - Family history of cardiovascular diseases
   - Sedentary lifestyle (lack of exercise)
   - Increased salt intake
   - Consumption of alcohol

Ans. 75. b 76. c 77. b 78. a

80. Dyspnea is often associated with:
    a. Left-sided heart failure
    b. Right-sided heart failure
    c. Atrial septal defect
    d. Ventricular septal defect

81. Chest pain is often a complaint of:
    a. Congenital heart diseases
    b. Hypertension
    c. Ischemic heart disease
    d. Hypotension

82. What are the terminologies used in describing cardiovascular diseases (CVDs)?

    The following are the terminologies used in describing cardiovascular diseases:
    - Ischemia: It is the local blockage or reduction of blood supply to a part of the myocardium.
    - Cardiac arrest: It refers to stoppage of beating of the heart.
    - Heart failure: It refers to inability of the heart to deliver the circulatory demands of the body.
    - Shock: Shock or hypotension refers to a reduction in the circulatory volume due to excessive bleeding or decreased venous return.

83. What are the signs and symptoms of cardiovascular diseases?

    The following are the signs and symptoms of cardiovascular diseases?
    - Dyspnea or breathlessness
    - Chest pain
    - Palpitation (awareness of the heart beat)
    - Cyanosis (bluish discolouration of the skin and mucous membrane
    - Edema (it is a feature of heart failure)
    - Orthopnea (breatlessness when the patient lies down flat)
    - Syncope (fainting or loss of consciousness due to reduction in the blood pressure
    - Blood pressure

Ans. 80. a 81. c

84. What are the causes for secondary hypertension?

There are various causes for secondary hypertension. These are the following:

- Cushing's syndrome
- Hyperaldosteronism
- Phaeochromocytoma
- Acromegaly
- Oral contraceptive and estrogen therapy
- Renal artery disease
- Glomerulonephritis
- Pyelonephritis
- Polycystic disease
- Renal artery stenosis
- Renal transplantation
- Nephropathy
- Cerebral edema due to cerebrovascular accidents, tumours or head injuries

85. Lateral pterygoid muscle is palpated at:
   a. Between superior and inferior temporal lines
   b. Maxillary tuberosity
   c. Ramus of mandible
   d. Lingual aspect of the mandible

86. For toluidine blue vital staining, what is the percentage of the stain used?
   a. 1 b. 2
   c. 3 d. 4

87. After applying toluidine blue vital stain, the area is irrigated with:
   a. Water b. Saline
   c. Acetic acid d. Alcohol

88. Among the following statements about toluidine blue vital staining test result, which is incorrect?
   a. It has an affinity for cells actively synthesizing nucleic acids
   b. Biopsy should be taken from site showing increased uptake
   c. Regenerating epithelium in the healing ulcers and dysplastic cells show uptake
   d. Keratotic lesions take up the dye

Ans. 85. b 86. b 87. c 88. d

89. The best biopsy method for salivary gland and cystic lesions is:
    a. Incisional biopsy
    b. Excisional biopsy
    c. Punch biopsy
    d. Fine needle aspiration cytology

90. Biopsy specimen obtained is preserved in:
    a. Alcohol
    b. Saline
    c. Water
    d. Formalin

91. What is the percentage of formalin used in the preservation of biopsy specimen?
    a. 1
    b. 10
    c. 20
    d. 90

92. Removal of surface cells for cytologic rxamination is called:
    a. FNAC
    b. Exfoliative cytology
    c. Punch biopsy
    d. Incisional biopsy

93. Among the following, which is used as a fixative in oral exfoliative cytology?
    a. Ethylene glycol
    b. Saline
    c. Xylene
    d. Paraaminobenzoic acid

94. In the interpretation of oral exfoliative cytology, Class III refers to:
    a. Cytology suggestive of malignancy but not definitely indicative
    b. Atypical cytology without any evidence of malignancy
    c. Normal cells
    d. Strongly suggestive of malignancy

95. What is the interpretation of oral exfoliative cytology?
    The oral exfoliative cytology is interpreted as given below:
    Class I : Normal cells
    Class II : Atypical cytology, and no evidence of malignancy
    Class III : Cytology suggestive of malignancy but not definitely indicative
    Class IV : Strongly suggestive of malignancy
    Class V : Conclusive for malignancy

Ans. 89. d 90. d 91. b 92. d 93. a 94. a

96. What is the normal pH of saliva?

a. 2.5–3.5 b. 4.0–5.0
c. 6.35–6.85 d. 6.95–7.25

97. Which biochemical value is increased in the saliva of children with cystic fibrosis?

a. Albumin b. Calcium
c. Phosphorus d. Nitrogen

98. Which biochemical value may be increased in the saliva of children with asthma?

a. Albumin b. Calcium
c. Phosphorus d. Nitrogen

99. Salivary ratio of which biochemical value is increased in Addison's disease?

a. Albumin and globulin
b. Sodium and potassium
c. Calcium and phosphorus
d. Magnesium and selenium

100. Salivary ratio of which biochemical value is decreased in Cushing's syndrome?

a. Albumin and globulin
b. Sodium and potassium
c. Calcium and phosphorus
d. Magnesium and selenium

Ans. 96. c 97. b 98. b 99. b 100. b

SECTION VIII

1. Salivary proteins and calcium may be elevated because of:
   a. Dehydration
   b. Starvation
   c. Stress following major surgical procedures
   d. Malnutrition

2. Which is the colour indicator used in Snyder test?
   a. Ziel-Nelson stain
   b. H & E stain
   c. Lugol's iodine
   d. Bromocresol green

3. Slivary buffer capacity is based on the presence of which chemical substance in the saliva?
   a. Glucose
   b. Calcium
   c. Bicarbonate
   d. Insulin

4. Serum hemoglobin is expressed as:
   a. Prcentage
   b. G/dl
   c. mg/dl
   d. Pico gram

5. Packed cell volume is also called as:
   a. Hemoglobin concentration
   b. Hematocrit
   c. Red cell index
   d. Mean corpuscular hemoglobin

6. Mean corpuscular volume is expressed as:
   a. Cubic microns
   b. Percentage
   c. µ g
   d. Cubic cm

7. Mean corpuscular hemoglobin concentration is expressed as:
   a. G/dl
   b. mg/dl
   c. Percentage
   d. Cubic microns

Ans. 1. c 2. d 3. c 4. b 5. b 6. a 7. c

8. How is mean corpuscular volume (MCV)calculated?

Mean corpuscular volume (MCV) is calculated using the formula:

$$MCV = \frac{\text{Hematocrit in percentage} \times 10}{\text{RBC count in millions/mm}^3}$$

It is expressed as cubic microns (μ^3)

9. What is the normal mean corpuscular volume?

a. $0.8 - 1.5\ \mu^3$
b. $12 - 18\ \mu^3$
c. $42 - 56\ \mu^3$
d. $82 - 100\ \mu^3$

10. How is mean corpuscular hemoglobin (MCH) calculated?

Mean corpuscular hemoglobin (MCH) is calculated using the formula:

$$MCH = \frac{\text{Hemoglobin in g/dl} \times 10}{\text{RBC count in million/mm}^3}$$

It is expressed as picogram (pg)

11. What is the normal value of mean corpuscular hemoglobin?

a. 0.2 – 3.8 mg
b. 10.1 – 18.5 μg
c. 26.0 – 34.0 pg
d. 30.0 – 110 IU

12. How is mean corpuscular hemoglobin concentration (MCHC) calculated?

$$MCHC = \frac{\text{Hemoglobin in g/dl} \times 100}{\text{Hematocrit in percentage}}$$

It is expressed as percentage

13. What is the normal value of mean corpuscular hemoglobin concentration?

a. 3.0 – 10.0 mg
b. 12.0 – 18 nanogram
c. 31.0 – 37.0%
d. 42.0 – 80.0 %

14. What is the normal hematocrit or packed cell volume?

a. 12.0 - 14.0 g
b. 38.0 - 50.0 per cent
c. 14.0 – 18.0 g
d. 34.0 – 56.0 per cent

Ans. 9. d 11. c 13. c 14. b

15. What is differential leukocyte cont (DLC)?

Differential leukocyte count (DLC) is expressed as average percentage of each cell type or as absolute numbers per volume of blood.

Cell Type	*Percentage*	*Absolute Number per mm³*
Neutrophils	43 to 77	3,000 to 7000
Basophils	0 to 2	0 to 100
Eosinophils	0 to 4	50 to 300
Lymphocytes	17 to 47	1,000 to 3,500
Monocytes	0 to 9	100 to 600

16. An increase in the number of immature neutrophils or bands more than 2 to 6 percent is described as:
    a. Shift to left
    b. Shift to right
    c. Shift to front
    d. Shift to back
17. Immature neutrophils appear in the peripheral blood due to:
    a. Allergy and parasitic infection
    b. Infections and bone marrow suppression
    c. Pregnancy and lactation
    d. Debilitating illnesses
18. A fall in the mature neutrophil count occurs in:
    a. Bone marrow suppression
    b. Allergic reaction
    c. Parasitic infection
    d. Anemia
19. Leukocytosis may occur in all of the following conditions, except:
    a. Infections
    b. Shock
    c. After excessive bleeding
    d. Immunosuppression
20. Which blood cell condition can occur in Addison's disease?
    a. Agranulocytosis
    b. Leukocytosis
    c. Eosinophilia
    d. Monocytosis
21. Lymphocytosis can occur in the following conditions, except:
    a. Allergy
    b. Lymphatic leukemia
    c. Infectious mononucleosis
    d. Convalescence from infections

Ans. 16. a 17. b 18. a 19. d 20. c 21. a

22. Monocytosis can occur in all the following conditions, except:
    a. Infective endocarditis
    b. Hodgkin's disease
    c. Malaria
    d. Infectious mononucleosis

23. Leukopenia can occur in all the following conditions, except:
    a. Typhoid fever
    b. Addison's disease
    c. Pernicious anemia
    d. Aleukemic leukemia

24. Cyclic neutropenia usually follows a cycle of:
    a. One week
    b. 3 days
    c. 21 days
    d. 45 days

25. What is pancytopenia and what are the causes?

    Pancytopenia refers to a fall in count of all the cellular elements of the blood. Following are the causes for pancytopenia:
    - Severe infectious conditions
    - Hemorrhage
    - Renal failure
    - Liver failure
    - Severe malnutrition
    - Radiation
    - Poisoning
    - Chemotherapy
    - Aplastic anemia
    - Iatrogenic (caused by certain drugs)

26. A peripheral blood smear examination helps in the determination of the following, except:
    a. Determining maturity
    b. Erythrocyte morphology
    c. Type of anemia
    d. Mean corpuscular hemoglobin

27. Anisocytosis is seen in:
    a. Iron deficiency anemia
    b. Pernicious anemia
    c. Megaloblastic anemia
    d. Sickle cell anemia

Ans. 22. d 23. b 24. c 26. d 27. a

28. Poikilocytosis is a feature of:
    a. Iron deficiency anemia
    b. Anemia due to blood loss
    c. Pernicious anemia
    d. Sickle cell anemia

29. An elevated erythrocyte sedimentation rate (ESR) is seen in all the following conditions, except:
    a. Inflammatory reactions
    b. Destructive tumours
    c. Lymphoma
    d. Polycythemia

29. A lowered erythrocyte sedimentation rate is seen in all the following conditions, except:
    a. Polycythemia
    b. Macrocytic hypochromic anemia
    c. Hemoglobinopathies
    d. Destructive tumours

30. What is the diameter of platelets?
    a. 0.2 – 0.4 microns
    b. 0.8 – 1.0 microns
    c. 2.0 – 4.0 microns
    d. 8.0 – 10.0 microns

31. Platelets may contain all the following, except:
    a. Serotonin
    b. Histamine
    c. Thromboplasin
    d. Acetylcholine

32. Platelets are also called as:
    a. X-cells
    b. Lymphoblasts
    c. Thrombocytes
    d. Blast cells

33. Capillary fragility test is performed in:
    a. Vitamin C deficiency
    b. Pernicious anemia
    c. Folic acid deficiency
    d. Iron deficiency

Ans. 28. c 29. d 30. c 31. d 32. c 33. d

34. Bleeding time (BT) is increased in the following conditions, except:
    a. Non-thrombocytopenic purpura
    b. Vitamin C deficiency
    c. Sickle cell anemia
    d. Severe infections

35. Defective clot retraction time generally indicates:
    a. Deficiency of Factor VIII
    b. Deficiency of Factor IX
    c. Qualitative and quantitative deficiency of platelets
    d. Vitamin C deficiency

36. Platelet activity is measured by:
    a. Nitroblue tetrazolium reduction test
    b. Break-up time
    c. Schilling's test
    d. Clot retraction time

37. Normal prothrombin time (PT) is:
    a. 2-6 minutes
    b. 3-5 seconds
    c. 11-15 seconds
    d. 25-45 seconds

38. Prothrombin time is prolonged in the deficiencies of following clotting Fcators except:
    a. I
    b. II
    c. III
    d. V

39. Prothrombin time may be increased due to:
    a. Anticoagulant therapy
    b. Immunosuppression
    c. Aplastic anemia
    d. Hypertension

40. Activated partial thromboplastin time (APTT) is helpful in the diagnosis of deficiency states of which clotting Factors?
    a. I and II
    b. III and IV
    c. VI and VII
    d. VIII and IX

Ans. 34. c 35. c 36. d 37. c 38. c 39. a 40. d

41. Clotting time is useful in determining:
    a. Anticoagulant activity
    b. Immunosuppression
    c. Aplastic anemia
    d. Hypertension

42. Chemical analysis is usually performed in:
    a. Whole blood
    b. Plasma
    c. Serum
    d. Blood concentrate

43. The main plasma proteins are the following, except:
    a. Albumin
    b. Globulin
    c. Fibrinogen
    d. Acetylcholine

44. Plasma proteins aid in the following functions, except:
    a. Maintenance of osmotic pressure
    b. Maintenance of buffering capacity
    c. Transport of hormones
    d. Chemotaxis

45. Normal serum protein level is:
    a. 04 – 1.8 mg/dl
    b. 1.0 – 2.5 mg/dl
    c. 6.0 – 8.0 g/dl
    d. 12.0 – 16.0 g/dl

46. The major constituent of serum protein is:
    a. Albumin
    b. Globulin
    c. Fibrinogen
    d. Thromboplastin

47. Albumin accounts for —— of serum proteins:
    a. 0.2 – 1.8 g/dl
    b. 1.0 – 2.0 g/dl
    c. 4.0 – 5.0 g/dl
    d. 8.0 – 12.0 g/dl

48. Low serum level of protein can occur in all the following conditions, except:
    a. Sprue
    b. Malnutrition
    c. Marasmus
    d. Addison's disease

Ans. 41. a 42. c 43. d 44. d 45. c 46. a 47. c 48. c

49. Increase in alpha globulin fraction of plasma proteins is seen in all the following conditions, except:

a. Carcinoma
b. Nephrosis
c. Cardiomyopathy
d. Rheumatic fever

50. Increase in gamma globulin fraction of plasma proteins occurs in all the following conditions, except:

a. Hepatitis
b. Cirrhosis
c. Lupus erythematosus
d. Rheumatic fever

51. Which are the conditions associated with increase in gamma globulin fraction of plasma proteins?

The following conditions are associated with increase in the gamma globulin fraction of the plasma proteins:

- Cirrhosis
- Hepatitis
- Lupus erythematosus
- Rheumatoid arthritis
- Multiple myeloma
- Sarcoidosis
- Myelogenous and monocytic leukemia
- Hodgkin's disease

52. What is the normal serum calcium level?

a. 9.0 – 11 mg/dl
b. 9.0 – 11 g/dl
c. 0.9 – 1.1 mg/dl
d. 0.9 – 1.1 g/dl

53. Which are the two forms of calcium present in the blood?

Calcium is present in two forms in the blood. These two forms are:

i. Protein-bound form
ii. Diffusible or ionizable form

54. Increase in serum calcium level is seen in all the following conditions, except:

a. Megaloblastic anemia
b. Polycythemia vera
c. Sarcoidosis
d. Primary hyperparathyroidism

Ans. 49. c 50. d 52. a 54. c

55. Hypocalcemia is seen in all the following conditions, except:
    a. Hypoparathyroidism
    b. Rickets
    c. Sarcoidosis
    d. Coeliac disease

56. What is the normal serum phosphorus level?
    a. 9.0 – 11 mg/dl
    b. 9.0 – 11 g/ dl
    c. 2.0 – 5.0 mg/dl
    d. 2.0 – 5.0 g/dl

57. Serum phosphorus level is decreased in the following conditions, except:
    a. Primary hyperparathyroidism
    b. Rickets
    c. Osteomalacia
    d. Sarcoidosis

58. Serum phosphorus level is increased in the following conditions, except:
    a. Hypoparathyroidism
    b. Renal insufficiency
    c. Hypervitaminosis D
    d. Osteomalacia

59. Serum alkaline phosphatase level is high in:
    a. Children
    b. Adults
    c. Postmenopausal women
    d. Pregnant women

60. Elevated serum alkaline phosphatase level is seen in all the following conditions, except:
    a. Paget's disease
    b. Osteomalacia
    c. Rickets
    d. Hypophosphatasia

61. Serum alkaline phosphatase level is lowered in all the following conditions, except:
    a. Osteomalacia
    b. Hypophosphatasia
    c. Scurvy
    d. Hypothyroidism

Ans. 55. c 56. d 57. d 58. d 59. a 60. d 61. a

62. Normal value of serum alkaline phosphatase level is:
    a. 10 – 40 Bodansky units
    b. 3 – 13 King-Armstrong units
    c. 13 – 25 International units
    d. 12.8 – 29.0 mg/dl

63. Among the following, which is suggestive of metastatic carcinoma of the prostate?
    a. Elevated serum alkaline phosphatase level
    b. Elevated acid phosphatase level
    c. Elevated serum uric acid level
    d. Elevated serum phosphorus level

64. Serum amylase leve is increased all the following conditions, except:
    a. Acute pancreatitis
    b. Mumps
    c. Sarcoidosis
    d. Intestinal obstruction

65. Uric acid is a by-product of:
    a. Carbohydrate metabolism
    b. Lipid metabolism
    c. Nucleoprotein metabolism
    d. Nitrogen metabolism

66. Increased level of uric acid may occur in the following conditions, except:
    a. Lymphoma
    b. Gout
    c. Acutc pancreatitis
    d. Lobar pneumonia

67. Normal value of serum uric acid is:
    a. 0.8 – 2.0 mg/dl
    b. 4.0 – 8.5 mg/dl
    c. 30.0 – 110 mg/dl
    d. 40.0 – 95.0 mg/dl

68. Serum uric acid level may be higher in:
    a. Males
    b. Females
    c. Children
    d. Neonates

Ans. 62. b 63. b 64. c 65. c 66. c 67. b 68. a

69. Serum cholesterol level may be higher in all the following conditions, except:
    a. Lymphoma
    b. Nephrotic syndrome
    c. Obese diabetic patients
    d. Hypothyroidism

70. Creatine phosphate dephosphorylation leading to the formation of creatine as metabolic product occurs in:
    a. Blood vessels
    b. Nerves
    c. Muscles
    d. Adipose tissue

71. Normal serum chloride level is:
    a. 12-25 m Eq/l
    b. 35 – 67 m Eq/l
    c. 25-42 m Eq/l
    d. 96 – 110 m Eq/l

72. Low serum alkaline phosphatase level is seen in all the following conditions, except:
    a. Rickets
    b. Hypophosphatasia
    c. Anemia
    d. Hypothyroidism

73. Increased level of serum alkaline phosphatase may be seen in all the following conditions, except:
    a. Osteomalacia
    b. Hypothyroidism
    c. Rickets
    d. Hyperparathyroidism

74. What is the normal value of serum alkaline phosphatase?
    Serum alkaline phosphatase level is expressed in three units. These are:
    - 1.0 – 4.0 Bodansky units
    - 3.0 – 13.0 King-Armstrong units (KA units)
    - 30.0 – 110.0 International Units (IU)

75. Serum sodium level may increase due to:
    a. Corticosteroid administration
    b. Dehydration
    c. Diseases of the kidney
    d. Addison's disease

76. What is the approximate percentage of total body iron present in hemoglobin?
    a. 10
    b. 30
    c. 60
    d. 90

Ans. 69. a 70. c 71. d 72. a 73. b 75. d 76. c

77. Serum iron refers to:
    a. Iron present in hemoglobin
    b. Iron bound to transferrin
    c. Iron present in liver
    d. Iron present in bone marrow

78. Normal serum iron level is:
    a. 0.5 – 1.8 μg/mm^3
    b. 5.5 – 18.5 μg/mm^3
    c. 55.0 – 185 μg/mm^3
    d. 0.05 – 018 μg/mm^3

79. Normal total iron-binding capacity is:
    a. 0.25 – 0.45 μg/mm^3
    b. 2.50 – 4.25 μg/mm^3
    c. 25.0 – 42.5 μg/mm^3
    d. 250.0 – 425.0 μg/mm^3

80. What is the significance of measuring serum enzymes?

    Serum enzymes are measured in suspected diseases involving various tissues and organ systems such as the following:
    - Myocardium
    - Liver
    - Pancreas
    - Megaloblastic anemia
    - Leukemia
    - Lymphoma

81. What is the other name for serum glutamic-oxaloacetic transaminase (SGOT)?
    a. Alkaline phosphatase
    b. Acid phosphatase
    c. Aspartate transaminase
    d. Uric acid

82. Aspartate transaminase and Alanine transaminase are present in the following tissues, except:
    a. Salivary gland
    b. Liver
    c. Heart
    d. Skeletal muscles

Ans. 77. b 78. c 79. d 81. c 82. a

83. Normal value of SGPT is:
    a. Below 0.25 U/litre
    b. Below 2.5 U/litre
    c. Below 25.0 U/litre
    d. Below 250.0 U/litre

84. Normal value of SGOT is:
    a. 0.8 – 5.0 U/litre
    b. 8.0 – 50 U/litre
    c. 80.0 – 500.0 U/litre
    d. 800.0 – 5000.U/litre

85. What is the normal value of lactate dehydrogenase (LDH)?
    a. 0.2 – 04 U/litre
    b. 2.0 – 4.0 U/litre
    c. 20.0 – 40 U/litre
    d. 200.0 – 400 U/litre

86. Lactate dehydrogenase (LDH) level is increased in the following conditions, except:
    a. Diseases of the myocardium
    b. Vitamin B12 and folic acid deficiency
    c. Pernicious anemia
    d. Chronic myelogenous leukemia

87. Which are the liver function tests (LFT)?

    Liver function tests are the following:
    - Serum bilirubin level
    - Urinary urobilinogen
    - Bromsulphalein (BSP) test
    - Serum cholesterol
    - Serum alkaline phosphatase
    - Lactate dehydrogenase (LDH)
    - Prothrombin time (PT)

88. What is the normal serum bilirubin level?
    a. 0 – 1.5 ¼g/dl
    b. 0 – 1.5 mg/dl
    c. 0 –1.5 U/dl
    d. 0 – 1.5 g/dl

89. Icterus refers to:
    a. Anemia
    b. Congenital deformities
    c. Absence of salivary gland
    d. Jaundice

Ans. 83. c 84. b 85. d 86. c 88. b 89. d

90. Serum bilirubin level may be increased in all the following conditions, except:
   a. Hemolytic anemia
   b. Hepatitis
   c. Cirrhosis
   d. Hemochromatosis

91. Among the following conditions, which is not associated with decreased urine output?
   a. Glomerulonephritis
   b. Congestive heart failure
   c. Diabetes insipidus
   d. Dehydration

92. Among the following conditions, which is not associated with increased urine output?
   a. Glomerulonephritis
   b. Diabetes mellitus
   c. Diabetes insipidus
   d. Diuretic therapy

93. Specific gravity of urine increases in all the following conditions, except:
   a. Excessive intake of water
   b. Dehydration
   c. Diabetes mellitus
   d. Nephrosis

94. Proteinuria is seen in all the following conditions, except:
   a. Multiple myeloma
   b. Nephrotic syndrome
   c. Infectious mononucleosis
   d. Macroblobulinemia

95. Normally, urine may contain the following, except:
   a. Epithelial cells
   b. Tyrosine
   c. Oxalate
   d. Phosphate

96. Which immunological test is useful in the diagnosis of rheumatoid arthritis?
   a. ELISA
   b. Western blot
   c. Immunofluorescence study
   d. Latex agglutination test

Ans. 90. d 91. c 92. a 93. a 94. c 95. b 96. d

97. Viral infections and syphilis can be diagnosed by which of the following tests?
    a. Agglutination test
    b. Complement fixation test
    c. Latex agglutination test
    d. Heterophil agglutination test

98. In heterophil agglutination test, RBCs obtained from —— are used?
    a. Pig
    b. Human beings
    c. Sheep
    d. Horse

99. Monospot test is used in the diagnosis of:
    a. Infectious mononucleosis
    b. AIDS
    c. Hepatitis B
    d. Systemic lupus erythematosus

100. Mazzini test is useful in the diagnosis of:
    a. Tuberculosis
    b. Hansen's disease
    c. Infectious mononucleosis
    d. Syphilis

Ans. 97. b 98. c 99. a 100. d

SECTION IX

1. Which are the immunofluorescent tests available?

   Immunofluorescence studies or fluorescent antibody tests are based on the principle that, a fluorescent dye (fluorescein) is used to couple the antibodies and then made to react with the specific antigens. The antigen-antibody reaction is observed microscopically (fluorescent microscopy).

   These tests are useful in the diagnosis of following lesions:

   - Pemphigus
   - Bullous pemphigoid
   - Benign mucous membrane (cicatricial) pemphigoid
   - Lupus erythematosus
   - Lichen planus

   Basically there are three types of immunofluorescent tests. These are:

   - Direct immunofluorescence tests
   - Indirect immunofluorescence tests
   - Sandwich technique

2. The reliable and confirmatory test for syphilis is:

   a. Dark-field microscopy b. VDRL test
   c. Wasserman reaction d. ELISA test

3. The following diseases may be associated with false positive results when serological tests for syphilis are carried out, except:

   a. Febrile diseases
   b. Measles
   c. Upper respiratory tract infections
   d. Viral fever

4. What is injected in Mantoux test?

   a. Mycobacterium tuberculosis
   b. Puified protein derivative
   c. Antibody
   d. Serum

Ans. 2. a 3. d 4. b

5. While performing patch test, the allergens are applied and the area is evaluated after:
   a. 24 to 48 hours
   b. After one week
   c. After 4 weeks
   d. After 72 hours

6. The basal metabolic rate (BMR) in a normal adult male is:
   a. 72 per minute
   b. 40 Cal./sq. M/hr
   c. 80 – 102 per minute
   d. 80 Cal./sq. M/hr

7. Normal plasma-bound iodine (PBI) ranges from:
   a. 0.2–0.8 μg/dl
   b. 4.0–8.0 μg/dl
   c. 12.0–19.0 μg/dl
   d. 40.0–80.0 μg/dl

8. Normal value of triiodothyronine uptake test is:
   a. 11–19 percent
   b. 21–29 percent
   c. 31–39 percent
   d. 41–49 percent

9. What is the normal value of serum thyroxin test?
   a. 0.4–1.1 μg/dl
   b. 4.0–11.0 μg/dl
   c. 40.0–110.0 μg/dl
   d. 400–1100 μg/dl

10. What is the fasting blood sugar level?
    a. 60–90 mg/dl
    b. 60–90 G/dl
    c. 90–120 mg/dl
    d. 90–120 G/dl

11. Benedict's test is carried out for determining:
    a. Blood urea level
    b. SGOT
    c. Urine sugar
    d. Basal metabolic rate (BMR)

12. "Brown tumour" refers to:
    a. Tumour involving the bone marrow
    b. Jaw lesions of hyperparathyroidism
    c. Osteogenic sarcoma
    d. Liver tumour

Ans. 5. a 6. b 7. b 8. a 9. b 10. a 11. c 12. b

13. Osteitis fibrosa cystica generalisata refers to the radiographic appearance of:
    a. Paget's disease
    b. Fibrous dysplasia
    c. Albright's syndrome
    d. Hyperparathyroidism jaw lesions

14. Vanillylmandelic acid assay (VMA) is carried out to assess:
    a. Bone maturation
    b. Adrenal function
    c. Renal function
    d. Salivary buffering capacity

15. Normal urinary vanillylmandelic acid assay (VMA) value is:
    a. 0.2 – 1.0 mg/24 hour urine sample
    b. 2.0 – 10 mg/24 hour urine sample
    c. 0.2 – 1.0 mg/1 hour urine sample
    d. 2.0 – 10 mg/1 hour urine sample

16. What is the sample that is used to do vanillylmandelic acid assay?
    a. Urine b. Serum
    c. Soft tissue d. Bone

17. What is the diagnostic test that is used in the diagnosis of Addison's disease?
    a. Wasserman reaction b. Kveim test
    c. Urinary 17-hydroxycorticosteroids
    d. Mono spot test

18. What are the clinical signs associated with disturbances of autonomic dysfunction?

    The following are the clinical signs associated with disturbances of autonomic dysfunction:
    - Flushing of the face
    - Blanching of the face
    - Hyperhidrosis
    - Anhidrosis
    - Ptosis or drooping of the eyelids
    - Miosis or dilatation of the pupils
    - Nasal congestion
    - Lacrimation
    - Alteration of saliva (qualitatively as well as quantitatively)

Ans. 13. d 14. b 15. b 16. a 17. c

19. What is the type of hepatitis B virus (HBV)?
    a. DNA virus
    b. RNA virus
    c. Both DNA and RNA virus
    d. Does not contain nucleic acid

20. What is the usual incubation period for hepatitis B virus infection?
    a. 1 – 6 months
    b. 1 – 6 weeks
    c. 1 – 6 days
    d. 1 – 6 years

21. Prodromal or preicteric phase of hepatitis B is characterized by:
    a. Flu-like symptoms
    b. Hepatomegaly
    c. Jaundice
    d. Splenomegaly

22. Icteric phase of hepatitis B is characterized by all the following, except:
    a. Jaundice
    b. Hepatomegaly
    c. Splenomegaly
    d. Flu-like symptoms

23. Complete recovery after hepatitis occurs within:
    a. One week
    b. One month
    c. Four months
    d. Four weeks

24. The icteric phase of hepatitis B lasts for:
    a. One week
    b. Four to six weeks
    c. Four to six months
    d. One month

25. Demonstration of Australia antigen is suggestive of:
    a. Hepatitis B
    b. Paget's disease
    c. Systemic lupus erythematosus
    d. Sarcoidosis

Ans. 19. a 20. a 21. a 22. d 23. c 24. b 25. a

26. Failure of HBsAg and HbeAg to seroconvert to anti-HBs and anti-Hbe is indicative of:
    a. Acute hepatitis B
    b. Acute hepatitis A
    c. Chronic hepatitis B
    d. Chronic hepatitis A

27. After treating a patient with hepatitis B, the non-autoclavable instruments must be sterilized by:
    a. Hot water sterilization
    b. 90% alcohol
    c. 2 per cent glutaraldehyde
    d. 0.2 per cent chlorhexidine gluconate

28. Multifocal vascular nodules in the skin and mucosa with a potential for dissemination into lymph nodes, gastrointestinal tract and lungs is called:
    a. Polyposis
    b. Fibromas
    c. Kawasaki disease
    d. Kaposi's sarcoma

29. The most common infection seen in AIDS patients is:
    a. Pharyngitis
    b. ANUG
    c. Candidiasis
    d. Pneumonia

30. The following features may be seen AIDS patients, except:
    a. Persistent diarrhea
    b. Thrombocytopenia
    c. Leukocytosis
    d. Weight loss

31. Elevation of which immunoglobulin may be seen in AIDS patients?
    a. IgA and IgG
    b. IgM and IgA
    c. IgD and IgM
    d. IgA and IgD

32. Western blot test is used in the diagnosis of:
    a. SLE
    b. AIDS
    c. Hepatitis B
    d. Sarcoidosis

Ans. 26. c 27. c 28. d 29. c 30. c 31. a 32. b

33. A high level of β_3 microglobulin is indicative of:
    a. Hepatitis B
    b. Development of AIDS
    c. Tuberculosis
    d. Metastasis of oral squamous cell carcinoma

34. Low counts of CD4 and T cell lymphocytes are suggestive of:
    a. Initial infection of AIDS
    b. Cure from AIDS
    c. Poor prognosis
    d. Low grade infection

35. P24 antigen in the blood is suggestive of:
    a. Oral squamous cell carcinoma
    b. SLE
    c. Hepatitis B
    d. AIDS

36. Radioimmunoprecipitation assay (RIPA) is used in the diagnosis of:
    a. AIDS
    b. Hepatitis A
    c. SLE
    d. DLE

37. Which is the test associated with identification of antibodies to specific viral proteins?
    a. ELISA
    b. Western blot
    c. Immunofluorescence assay (IFA)
    d. Radioimmunoprecipitation assay (RIPA)

38. Zidovudine is a drug used in the treatment of:
    a. Hepatitis B
    b. Epilepsy
    c. Trigeminal neuralgia
    d. AIDS

39. What is the most serious toxic effect of zidovudine therapy?
    a. Hypersensitivity
    b. Generalized lymphadenopathy
    c. Bone marrow suppression
    d. Nephrotoxicity

Ans. 33. b 34. c 35. d 36. a 37. d 38. d 39. c

40. Interferon-α has been used to treat which condition associated with AIDS?

    a. Pneumocystis carinii pneumonia
    b. Kaposi's sarcoma
    c. Tuberculosis
    d. Candidiasis

41. Difficulty in breathing while lying down is called:

    a. Apnea
    b. Dyspnea
    c. Orthopnea
    d. None of the above

42. The cause for orthopnea may be:

    a. Rise in pressure of right atrium and right ventricle
    b. Rise in pressure of left atrium and left venticle
    c. Rise in pressure in right atrium and left ventricle
    d. Rise in pressure in left atrium and right ventricle

43. Pedal edema is indicative of:

    a. Lung disease
    b. Heart failure
    c. Thrombophlebitis
    d. Congenital heart disease

44. Palpitation may be associated with all the following conditions, except:

    a. Anxious persons
    b. Paroxysmal tachycardia
    c. Atrial fibrillation
    d. Decreased peripheral resistance

45. Among the following, which is not a cause for syncope?

    a. Decreased cardiac output
    b. Increased peripheral resistance
    c. Stress
    d. Prolonged standing

46. Among the following, which may not be a cardiac cause for syncope?

    a. Coronary artery disease
    b. Aortic stenosis
    c. Hypertrophic cardiomyopathy
    d. Dspnea

Ans. 40. b 41. c 42. a 43. b 44. d 45. b 46. d

47. Anemia is best checked in:
    a. Lower palpebral conjunctiva
    b. Bulbar conjunctiva
    c. Soft palate
    d. Fingers

48. Peripheral cyanosis may be caused by all the following, except:
    a. Vasoconstriction
    b. Low cardiac output
    c. Stress
    d. Vasodilatation

49. The first heart sound occurs due to:
    a. Closure of the aortic valve
    b. Closure of the mitral valve
    c. Closure of the pulmonary valve
    d. Contraction of the atrium

50. Heart murmurs may be heard in the following conditions, except:
    a. Anemia
    b. Pregnancy
    c. Abnormal heart valves
    d. Hyperparathyroidism

51. On a physiological basis, arterial blood pressure is a function of the following components, except:
    a. Cardiac output
    b. Intravascular fluid volume
    c. Extravascular fluid volume
    d. Peripheral vascular resistence

52. In the type of hypertension (HT), if the cause is unknown it is called:
    a. Essential HT
    b. Secondary hypertension
    c. Physiological hypertension
    d. Iatrogenic hypertension

53. Among the following, which may not be a cause for secondary hypertension?
    a. Renal diseases
    b. Atherosclerosis
    c. Cushing's disease
    d. Bronchitis

Ans. 47. a 48. d 49. b 50. d 51. c 52. a 53. d

54. In a hypertensive patient, blood investigation is mainly done for the following, except:
    a. Plasma rennin activity
    b. Urinary metanephrine
    c. Glucose
    d. 17-ketosteroids

55. In antihypertensive therapy, which is not included?
    a. Diuretics
    b. Plasma dilators
    c. Calcium channel blockers
    d. Combination of diuretic and non-diuretic drugs

56. Among the following, which is not a feature of rheumatic fever?
    a. Tachycardia
    b. Weight gain
    c. Joint pain, swelling and stiffness
    d. Fatigue

57. The major criteria in Duckett Jones' criteria for rheumatic fever does not include:
    a. Carditis
    b. Arhritis
    c. Arthralgia
    d. Chorea

58. The minor criteria in Duckett Jones' criteria for rheumatic fever does not include:
    a. Fever
    b. Arthralgia
    c. Subcutaneous nodules
    d. Increased ESR

59. Using Duckett Jones' criteria, rhematic fever is diagnosed based on:
    a. One major and one minor criteria or two major and one minor criteria
    b. Two major or one major and two minor criteria
    c. Two major and three minor criteria or one major and three minor criteria
    d. One major and three minor criteria or two major and two minor criteria

---

Ans. 54. c 55. b 56. b 57. c 58. c 59. b

60. In rheumatic fever, the antistreptolysin 'O' titre is usually above:
    a. 0.3 Todd units
    b. 30 Todd units
    c. 300 Todd units
    d. 3000 Todd units

61. Among the following, which may not be a cause for coronary heart disease?
    a. Coronary atheroasclerosis
    b. Dissecting aneurysms
    c. Carbon monoxide poisoning
    d. Diabetes insipidus

62. What are the causes assoiciated with coronary heart disease?

    The coronary artery diseases are angina pectoris and myocardial infarction. The following are the causes for coronary heart disease:
    - Atherosclerosis involving coronary blood vessels
    - Spasm of the coronary arteries
    - Aortic valvular disease
    - Dissecting aneurysms
    - Acute anemia
    - Carbon monoxide poisoning
    - Tachycardia

63. Stable angina differs from unstable angina in that?
    a. Here the cause is known
    b. Relieved by rest
    c. Relieved by sublingual nitroglycerine
    d. Does not respond to any medication

64. An attack of angina, when it exceeds how much time is called myocardial infarction?
    a. 10 seconds
    b. 30 seconds
    c. 3 minutes
    d. 5 minutes

65. The common complications of myocardial infarction are:
    a. Cardiac arrhythmias and congestive heart failure
    b. Heart failure and renal disease
    c. Chronic obstructive pulmonary disease
    d. Hypertension and renal failure

Ans. 60. c 61. d 63. b 64. b 65. a

66. The clinical features of myocardial infarction do not include:
   a. Chest pain
   b. Pain persisting more than 30 seconds
   c. Pain is relieved by sublingual nitroglycerine administration
   d. Radiation of pain to the left arm or left jaw

67. Chest pain associated with myocardial infarction is relieved by:
   a. Sublingual administration of nitroglycerine
   b. Aspirin
   c. Morphine sulphate
   d. Ibuprofen

68. Cardiac arrhythmia is often associated with:
   a. Smoking
   b. Atherosclerotic heart disease
   c. Congenital heart disease
   d. Angina pectoris

69. Where are Osler's nodes seen?
   a. Finger tips
   b. Body of the mandible
   c. Buccal surface of maxillary first molar
   d. In the developing alveolus of the newborn

70. Among the following investigations, which is not required for the evaluation of infective endocarditis?
   a. Blood culture
   b. Kveim test
   c. Plasma alkaline phosphatase
   d. Platelet count

71. What is the percentage of incidence of congenital heart diseases?
   a. 0.1%   b. 1%
   c. 10%   d. 0.8%

72. Children with congenital heart disease usually manifest the following, except:
   a. Breathlessness
   b. Inability to thrive
   c. Cyanosis
   d. Mental retardation

Ans. 66. c 67. c 68. b 69. a 70. b 71. b 72. d

73. Cyanosis is usually the result of:
    a. Entry of deoxygenated blood in the systemic circulation
    b. Entry of oxygenated blood in the systemic circulation
    c. Entry of deoxygenated blood in the portal circulation
    d. Entry of oxygenated blood in the portal circulation

74. What is the probable etiological factor suggested for congenital heart diseases?
    a. Maternal HIV infection
    b. Smoking during pregnancy
    c. Antibiotic therapy during pregnancy
    d. Maternal rubella infection

75. The condition wherein there is recirculation of blood through the lungs due to arteriovenous shunts is called:
    a. Coarctation of aorta
    b. Persistent ductus arteriosus
    c. Atrial septal defect
    d. Pulmonary stenosis

76. Clinical features such as headaches, cardiac symptoms, weakness or cramps of the legs, arterial pulsations of the neck and systolic murmur are features of:
    a. Persistent ductus arteriosus
    b. Coarctation of aorta
    c. Atrial septal defect
    d. Ventricular septal defect

77. Progressive enlargement of the right side of the heart and the pulmonary artery with its branches are features of:
    a. Persistent ductus arteriosus
    b. Coarctation of aorta
    c. Atrial septal defect
    d. Ventricular septal defect

78. Pulmonary vascular damage and heart failure are features of severe case of:
    a. Persistent ductus arteriosus
    b. Coarctation of aorta
    c. Atrial septal defect
    d. Ventricular septal defect

Ans. 73. a 74. d 75. b 76. d 77. c 78. d

79. Among the following statements about pulmonary stenosis, which is incorrect?
    a. It can occur alone as an isolated abnormality
    b. It can occur along with atrial septal defect
    c. It can occur along with ventricular septal defect
    d. It can occur in association with persistent ductus arteriosus

80. Fallot's tetralogy refers to:
    a. Pulmonary stenosis with coarctation of aorta
    b. Ventricular septal defect with persistent ductus arteriosus
    c. Pulmonary stenosis with ventricular septal defect
    d. Ventricular septal defect with coarctation of aorta

81. Fallot's tetralogy does not include:
    a. Persistent ductus arteriosus
    b. Pulmonary stenosis
    c. Ventricular septal defect
    d. Dextroposition of aorta

82. Among the following etiological factors, which may not be associated with vasovagal syncope?
    a. Emotional stress
    b. Prolonged standing
    c. Hyperglycemia
    d. Hyperventilation

83. What are the causes for syncope?

    Syncope refers to a temporary circulatory insufficiency. Following are the factors responsible for syncope:

    - Emotional stress
    - Standing for a long period of time
    - Hunger
    - Decreased blood sugar level (hypoglycemia)
    - Hyperventilation
    - Diseases of the heart
    - Loss of fluids excessively
    - Inadequate venous return (referred to as venous stasis)
    - Decreased cardiac output
    - Improper oxygenation of the blood
    - Disorders affecting the central nervous system (CNS)

Ans. 79. d 80. c 81. a 82. c

84. Among the following, which is not an example for diseases of the lower respiratory tract?
    a. Bronchial asthma
    b. Acute bronchitis
    c. Histoplasmosis
    d. Pharyngitis

85. Acute coryza refers to:
    a. Allergy to drugs
    b. Common cold
    c. Viral infection affecting the oral mucous membrane
    d. Bacterial infection causing salivary gland enlargement

86. Laryngitis may be associated with the following, except:
    a. Acute coryza
    b. Measles
    c. Excessive use of vocal cords
    d. Histoplasmosis

87. Radiographic features of translucent lung fields, bullae, low flat diaphragm and prominence of pulmonary hilar arterial shadows are features of:
    a. Tuberculosis
    b. Emphysema
    c. Bronchitis
    d. Secondaries in the lungs

88. Among the following statements about the dental considerations of bronchial asthma, which is wrong?
    a. NSAIDs are contraindicated
    b. Patients are more prone for nasopharyngeal candidiasis because of the use of corticosteroid inhalers
    c. Rubber dam isolation during dental treatment is necessary
    d. Some of the bronchodilators can cause xerostomia

89. The most important clinical feature of emphysema is:
    a. Cyanosis
    b. Clubbing
    c. Exertional dyspnea
    d. Anemia

90. Hypertrophy and hypersecretion of the mucous glands of the bronchial tree forming mucous plugs which block the airways are features of:
    a. Chronic bronchitis
    b. Emphysema
    c. Bronchiolitis
    d. Tuberculosis

Ans. 84. d 85. b 86. d 87. b 88. c 89. c 90. a

91. Presence of cough at least three months during two consecutive years is diagnostic of:
   a. Emphysema
   b. Chronic bronchitis
   c. Bronchiolitis
   d. Pulmonary tuberculosis

92. Diminished pulmonary function gradually leading to increased pulmonary resistance, ultimately leading to right-sided heart failure (cor pulmonale) are features of:
   a. Emphysema
   b. Bronchiolitis
   c. Chronic bronchitis
   d. Pulmonary tuberculosis

93. Use of adrenaline in local anesthetic agent in patients with cor pulmonale can result in:
   a. Bronchospasm
   b. Bronchoconstriction
   c. Cardiac arrhythmia
   d. Bronchial edema

94. Mucoviscidosis is also called as:
   a. Cellulitis
   b. Cystic fibrosis
   c. Mucositis
   d. Mucous patches

95. Blockage of pancreatic ducts by mucus leading to pancreatic insufficiency is a feature of:
   a. Bronchial asthma
   b. Cystic fibrosis
   c. Cirrhosis of liver
   d. Right heart failure

96. Dysphagia may be associated with the following, except:
   a. Myasthenia gravis
   b. Myotonic dystrophy
   c. Scleroderma
   d. Cystic fibrosis

Ans. 91. b 92. c 93. c 94. b 95. b 96. d

97. Retrosternal pain or burning sensation may be features of:
    a. Esophageal ulcers
    b. Intestinal ulcers
    c. Gastric ulcers
    d. Crohn's disease

98. Characteristic epigastric pain occurring before food intake or a few hours after food intake is a feature of:
    a. Duodenal ulcers
    b. Esophageal ulcers
    c. Gastric ulcers
    d. Peptic ulcers

99. The causes for cirrhosis of the liver may be the following, except:
    a. Hemochromatosis
    b. Wilson's disease
    c. Primary biliary cirrhosis
    d. Sarcoidosis

100. Lupus vulgaris refers to:
    a. Skin lesions of tuberculosis
    b. Complication of acute necrotizing ulcerative gingivostomatitis
    c. Lesions of syphilis
    d. Oral manifestation of systemic lupus erythematosus

Ans. 97. a 98. a 99. d 100. a

SECTION X

1. In the clotting mechanism, conversion of fibrinogen to fibrin is done by:
   a. Ionic calcium
   b. Tissue thromboplastin
   c. Thrombin
   d. Platelets
2. In the clotting mechanism, insoluble fibrin Ib is precipitated by:
   a. Ionic calcium
   b. Factor VIII
   c. Factor XIII a
   d. Factor IX
3. Inactive prothrombin is converted to thrombin by:
   a. Thromboplastin
   b. Ionic calcium
   c. Factor VIII
   d. Factor XI
4. Whiat is the name of Factor I?
   a. Prothrombin
   b. Fibrinogen
   c. Tissue thromboplastin
   d. Labile factor
5. The other name of Factor VIII is:
   a. Plasma thromboplastin
   b. Anti-hemophilic globulin
   c. Christmas Factor
   d. Prothrombin
6. The adherence of the platelets with each other takes place with the help of:
   a. Ionic calcium   b. ADP
   c. ATP   d. Tissue Factor

Ans. 1. c   2. c   3. a   4. b   5. b   6. b

7. If the blood vessels are intact, the platelets do not adhere probably because of the presence of:
   a. Factor VIII
   b. Fibrinogen
   c. Prostaglandin
   d. Clot retraction factors
8. Chemically, fibrinogen is:
   a. Lipid
   b. Carbohydrate
   c. Glycoprotein
   d. Collagen
9. The normal bleeding time is:
   a. 11–15 seconds
   b. Less than 2 minutes
   c. 5–10 minutes
   d. 20–30 minutes
10. Increased bleeding time is suggestive of:
    a. Calcium deficiency
    b. Factor VIII deficiency
    c. Platelet abnormalities
    d. Factor XI deficiency
11. Among the investigations for bleeding disorders, which one of the following is not included?
    a. Ascorbic acid assay
    b. Platelet survival time
    c. Prothrombin time
    d. Determination of blood pressure
12. Normal prothrombin time (PT) is:
    a. 5–10 minutes
    b. 11–15 seconds
    c. 20 minutes
    d. 40 seconds
13. Normal partial thromboplastin time is:
    a. 11–15 seconds
    b. 5–10 minutes
    c. 25–40 seconds
    d. 20 seconds
14. Normal blood coagulation time is:
    a. 5 minutes
    b. Less than 5 minutes
    c. 11–15 seconds
    d. 10–25 minutes

Ans. 7. c 8. c 9. c 10. d 11. d 12. b 13. c 14. d

15. Platelet survival time is determined in case of:
    a. Thrombocytopenic purpura
    b. Hemophilia
    c. Christmas disease
    d. Von Willebrand's disease

16. The normal platelet survival time is:
    a. Less than 5 minutes
    b. 1–2 weeks
    c. 8–9 days
    d. 3 months

17. Capillary fragility test is indicated in:
    a. Hemophilia
    b. Vitamin C deficiency
    c. Diabetes mellitus
    d. Hypertension

18. Among the following features of hemophilia, which is wrong?
    a. Episodes of hematuria
    b. Hemarthrosis
    c. Bleeding from small cuts and abrasions
    d. Increased bleeding time

19. The coagulation time is normal if Factor VIII activity is:
    a. Above 2 per cent
    b. Above 0.2 per cent
    c. Above 20 per cent
    d. Above 30 per cent

20. Hemohilia is managed by:
    a. Platelet transfusion
    b. Fresh whole blood transfusion
    c. Transfusion of serum
    d. Transfusion of RBCs

21. The advantage of using cryoprecipitate in the management of hemophilia is:
    a. It provides higher levels of AHG
    b. It is more stable than plasma
    c. It contains more ionic calcium
    d. It can be frozen

Ans. 15. a 16. c 17. b 18. d 19. a 20. b 21. a

22. Each pack of cryoprecipitate increases the level of Factor VIII by:
    a. 3.5 per cent
    b. 7.5 per cent
    c. 10.5 per cent
    d. 12.5 per cent
23. Epsilon aminocaproic acid (EACA) is used in case of:
    a. During endodontic treatment for calcified canals
    b. Hemophilia
    c. Lichen planus
    d. Leukoplakia
24. Plasminogen activity can be diminished by:
    a. Factor VIII
    b. Vitamin C
    c. Tranexamic acid
    d. Cryoprecipitate
25. Christmas disease refers to a deficiency state of which clotting Factor?
    a. VII
    b. VIII
    c. IX
    d. X
26. Which vitamin is required for the synthesis of prothrombin?
    a. A
    b. C
    c. E
    d. K
27. Treatment of idiopathic thrombocytopenic purpura is by:
    a. Aspirin
    b. Vitamin C
    c. Methotrexate
    d. Corticosteroids
28. Schönlein-Henoch syndrome is also called as:
    a. Idiopathic thrombocytopenic purpura
    b. Anaphylactoid purpura
    c. Thrombasthenia
    d. Symptomatic thrombocytopenic purpura
29. Among the following features of Ehlers-Danlos syndrome, which is incorrect?
    a. There can be prolonged bleeding after extraction
    b. There can be subcutaneous nodules (fat lobules)
    c. There can be pseudotumours
    d. There can be hypomobility of the joints

Ans. 22. a 23. b 24. c 25. c 26. d 27. d 28. b 29. d

30. Rendu-Weber-Osler syndome is also called as:
    a. Idiopathic thrombocytopenic purpura (ITP)
    b. Anaphylactoid purpura
    c. Hereditary hemorrhagic telangiectasia
    d. Thrombasthenia

31. The treatment modality available for hereditary hemorrhagic telangiectasia is:
    a. Radiotherapy
    b. Chemotherapy
    c. Cautery excision
    d. Sclerosing the lesion

32. Polycythemia rubra vera is characterized by:
    a. Neoplastic proliferation of RBCs
    b. Abnormally shaped RBCs
    c. RBCs with less hemoglobin content
    d. RBCs with sickle shape

33. One of the treatment modality available for treating polycythemia rubra vera is:
    a. Aspirin administration
    b. Use of methotrexate
    c. Phlebotomy
    d. Radiotherapy

34. "Angry appearance" is a feature of:
    a. Paget's disease
    b. Fibrous dysplasia
    c. Polycythemia rubra vera
    d. Discoid lupus erythematosus

35. Oral administration of triethylenemelamine is indicated in the treatment of:
    a. Myasthenia gravis
    b. Polycythemia rubra vera
    c. Trigeminal neuralgia
    d. Systemic lupus erythematosus

Ans. 30. c 31. c 32. a 33. c 34. c 35. b

36. Which condition is associated with RBC count as high as 10 million/ mm^3?
    a. Plummer Vinson syndrome
    b. Chronic myeloid leukemia
    c. Sickle cell anemia
    d. Polycythemia rubra vera
37. Iron-deficiency anemia is diagnosed by the following, except:
    a. Lowered Hb count
    b. Increased MCH, MCHC and MCV
    c. Low serum iron and decreased concentration of ferritin
    d. Microcytic hypochromic erythrocytes
38. In case of iron-deficiency anemia, iron supplements may be required for:
    a. 3 days
    b. 3 weeks
    c. 3 months
    d. 3 years
39. Plummer-Vinson syndrome does not include:
    a. Stomatitis
    b. Dysphagia
    c. Koilonychia
    d. Sickling of RBCs
40. Schilling's test is indicated in the diagnosis of:
    a. Vitamin B_{12} deficiency
    b. Iron deficiency anemia
    c. Sickle cell anemia
    d. Vitamin C deficiency
41. What specimen is used in performing Schilling's test?
    a. Saliva
    b. Serum
    c. Urine
    d. Whole blood
42. Lack of gastric intrinsic factor can result in which type of anemia?
    a. Sickle cell
    b. Iron deficiency
    c. Aplastic
    d. Pernicious
43. Neurological symptoms are associated with which type of anemia?
    a. Aplastic
    b. Folic acid deficiency
    c. Pernicious
    d. Plummer-Vinson syndrome

Ans. 36. d 37. b 38. c 39. d 40. a 41. c 42. d 43. c

44. What is supplemented in the management of pernicious anemia?
   a. Iron
   b. Folic acid
   c. Vitamin C
   d. Vitamin A

45. Oral manifestations of folic acid deficiency anemia may be the following, except:
   a. Angular cheilitis
   b. Ulcerative stomatitis
   c. Esophageal webs
   d. Pharyngitis

46. Aplastic anemia is caused by:
   a. Deficiency of iron
   b. Deficiency of gastric intrinsic factor
   c. Excessive hemolysis
   d. Bone marrow suppression

47. Fanconi's anemia and dyskeratosis congenita can lead to:
   a. Aplastic anemia
   b. Iron deficiency anemia
   c. Pernicious anemia
   d. Folic acid deficiency anemia

48. Among the following, which may not be a cause for aplastic anemia?
   a. Chloramphenicol
   b. Steroids
   c. Sulphonamides
   d. Benzene

49. Androgenic steroids may be indicated in the treatment of:
   a. Aplastic anemia
   b. Pernicious anemia
   c. Folic acid deficiency anemia
   d. Plummer-Vinson syndrome

50. Among the following, which may not be a cause for anemia?
   a. Infectious diseases
   b. Connective tissue diseases
   c. Leukemia
   d. Hyperthyroidism

Ans. 44. b 45. c 46. d 47. a 48. b 49. a 50. d

51. Pseudohemophilia refers to:
    a. Christmas disease
    b. Vitamin C deficiency
    c. Idiopathic thrombocytopenic purpura
    d. Von Willebrand's disease

52. Von Willebrand's disease is characterized by the following:
    a. Improper contraction of the capillaries with AHG deficiency
    b. AHG deficiency and platelet deficiency
    c. Normal AHG and abnormal capillary contraction
    d. Platelet deficiency and abnormal capillary contraction

53. Among the following hemorrhagic disorders, which may be associated with angioneurotic edema?
    a. ITP
    b. Thrombocytopathy
    c. Hemophilia
    d. Anaphylactoid purpura

54. Henoch's purpura is usually associated with:
    a. Joint pains
    b. Abdominal colic
    c. Ecchymosis
    d. Epistaxis

55. Hereditary hemorrhagic telangiectasia can affect the following surfaces, except:
    a. Cutaneous
    b. Visceral
    c. Muscle
    d. Mucosal

56. Among the following, which is not a sickle cell disease?
    a. Heterozygous sickle cell trait
    b. Homozygous sickle cell anemia
    c. Heterozygous sickling associated with hemoglobinopathy
    d. Homozygous sickling associated with hemoglobinopathy

57. Sickle cell anemia is characterized by all the following, except:
    a. Polycythemia
    b. Jaundice
    c. Growth retardation
    d. Skeletal abnormalities

Ans. 51. d 52. a 53. d 54. b 55. c 56. d 57. a

58. "Step-ladder" pattern of alveolar bone on radiographic examination is a feature of:

    a. Aplastic anemia
    b. Thalassemia
    c. Plummer-Vinson syndrome
    d. Sickle cell anemia

59. "Hair-on-end appearance on radiographic appearance is a feature of:

    a. Aplastic anemia
    b. Pernicious anemia
    c. Sickle cell disease
    d. Folic acid deficiency anemia

60. Demonstration of sickling is done with the help of:

    a. Sodium citrate
    b. EDTA
    c. Sodium meta bisulphate
    d. Stannous chloride

61. What is the percentage of sodium metabisulphate used to demonstrate sickling?

    a. 0.1 b. 1.0
    c. 10.0 d. 100.0

62. Sickle cell disease is treated with:

    a. Methotrexate
    b. Steroids
    c. Immunomodulators
    d. None of the above

63. Aplastic crisis is associated with:

    a. Pernicious anemia
    b. Sickle cell disease
    c. ITP
    d. Folic acid deficiency anemia

64. Abnormal hemoglobin chain associated with excessive production and accumulation of unaffected chain within the erythrocytes is a feature of:

    a. Sickle cell disease b. Aplastic anemia
    c. Pernicious anemia d. Thalassemia

Ans. 58. d 59. c 60. c 61. c 62. d 63. b 64. d

65. Cooley's anemia is also called as:
   a. Thalassemia major
   b. Thalassemia minor
   c. Aplastic anemia
   d. Pernicious anemia
66. Cyclic neutropenia usually follows a cycle of:
   a. 3 days
   b. 1 week
   c. 2 weeks
   d. 3 weeks
67. Cyclic neutropenia can be diagnosed by:
   a. Complete blood count
   b. Differential leukocyte count
   c. Repeated WBC count
   d. Clinical picture
68. Inability of the leukocytes to migrate from the bone marrow to the peripheral blood is called:
   a. Lazy leukocyte syndrome
   b. Cyclic neutropenia
   c. Agranulocytosis
   d. Chédiak-Higashi syndrome
69. Patients with lazy leukocyte syndrome are more prone for:
   a. Gingivitis and periodontitis
   b. Abscesses and cellulitis of dental origin
   c. Pulmonary infections and otitis media
   d. Osteomyelitis
70. The basic pathology of Chédiak-Higashi syndrome is:
   a. Abnormally shaped WBCs
   b. Presence of abnormal granules in the granulocytes and melanocytes
   c. Abnormal movement of WBCs to the site of infection
   d. Excessive proliferation of WBCs
71. Among the following statements about Chédiak-Higashi syndrome, which is incorrect?
   a. It is characterized by presence of abnormal granules in the granulocytes and melanocytes
   b. Neutrophils exhibit lack of chemotactic and bactericidal function
   c. There is inability to phagocytose the pathogens
   d. It may be due to impaired lysosomal activity of the granule-containing cells

---

Ans. 65. a 66. d 67. c 68. a 69. c 70. b 71. c

72. Improper pigmentation of skin and hair and recurrent infections involving skin and respiratory tract usually caused by gram-positive organisms are features of:
    a. Agranulocytosis
    b. Chédiak-Higashi syndrome
    c. Lazy leukocyte syndrome
    d. Cyclic neutropenia

73. Alternate-day corticosteroid therapy is indicated in which condition?
    a. Cyclic neutropenia
    b. Chédiak-Higashi syndrome
    c. Chronic idiopathic neutropenia
    d. Leukemia

74. Which type of leukemia is more prevalent in children?
    a. Acute lymphoblastic leukemia
    b. Acute non-lymphoblastic leukemia
    c. Chronic lymphocytic leukemia
    d. Chronic myeloid leukemia

75. Reticulum cell sarcoma is also known as:
    a. Histiocytic lymphoma
    b. Non-Hodgkin's lymphoma
    c. Hodgkin's disease
    d. Burkitt's lymphoma

76. Which is the most rapidly progressing jaw tumour?
    a. Squamous cell carcinoma
    b. Burkitt's lymphoma
    c. Basal cell carcinoma
    d. Adenomatoid odontogenic tumour

77. Rubbery consistency of the lymph nodes are typical of:
    a. Infections
    b. Malignancy
    c. Lymphoma
    d. Lipoma

78. Pel-Ebstein fever is characteristically seen in case of:
    a. Hodgkin's disease
    b. Non-Hodgkin's lymphoma
    c. Burkitt's lymphoma
    d. Histiocytic lymphoma

Ans. 72. b 73. c 74. a 75. a 76. b 77. c 78. a

79. Ann Arbor staging is done for:
    a. Hodgkin's disease
    b. Non-Hodgkin's lymphoma
    c. Burkitt's lymphoma
    d. Histiocytic lymphoma

80. Among the following histologic types of Hodgkin's disease, which has the worst prognosis?
    a. Lymphocyte predominant
    b. Lymphocyte depleted
    c. Nodular sclerosing
    d. Mixed cellularity

81. Among the following histologic types of Hodgkin's disease, which one has the best prognosis?
    a. Lymphocyte predominant
    b. Lymphocyte depleted
    c. Nodular sclerosing
    d. Mixed cellularity

82. Burkitt's lymphoma affects which part of the mandible more commonly?
    a. Incisor region
    b. Molar region
    c. Premolar region
    d. Canine region

83. Multiple punched out radiolucent areas are characteristic of:
    a. Hyperparathyroidism
    b. Multiple myeloma
    c. Histiocytic lymphoma
    d. Burkitt's lymphoma

84. Presence of Bence Jones protein in the urine is suggestive of:
    a. Diabetes mellitus
    b. Histiocytic lymphoma
    c. Hyperparathyroidism jaw lesions
    d. Multiple myeloma

85. Among the following, loss of lamina dura on radiographic examination may be a feature of:
    a. Multiple myeloma
    b. Burkitt's lymphoma
    c. Hodgkin's disease
    d. Non-Hodgkin's lymphoma

Ans. 79. a 80. b 81. a 82. b 83. b 84. d 85. a

86. The diagnostic test for multiple myeloma is:
    a. ANA test
    b. RIPA test
    c. Bence Jones proteins in the urine
    d. Mono spot test

87. Amyloid-like deposition in the gingiva and tongue can occur in:
    a. Multiple myeloma
    b. Histiocytic lymphoma
    c. Non-Hodgkin's lymphoma
    d. Hodgkin's disease

88. Apex of the maxillary sinus is formed by:
    a. Lateral wall of the nose
    b. Alveolus
    c. Zygomatic process of the maxilla
    d. Floor of the orbit

89. Roof of the maxillary sinus is formed by:
    a. Lateral wall of the nose
    b. Alveolus
    c. Zygomatic process of the maxilla
    d. Floor of the orbit

90. The shape of the maxillary sinus is:
    a. Oval
    b. Rhomboidal
    c. Pyramidal
    d. Rectangular

91. Among the following, which may not be a function of the maxillary sinus?
    a. It adds resonance to the voice
    b. It adds to the heaviness of the skull
    c. It warms the inspired air
    d. It adds moisture to the inspired air

92. In normal condition, the thickness of the mucosal lining of the maxillary sinus is:
    a. 1 mm
    b. 3 mm
    c. 5 mm
    d. 10 mm

93. The average volume of the maxillary sinus is:
    a. 0.5 ml
    b. 1.0 ml
    c. 7.0 ml
    d. 15.0 ml

Ans. 86. c 87. a 88. c 89. d 90. c 91. b 92. a 93. d

94. Among the following, which may not be a radiographic feature of maxillary sinusitis?
    a. Thinning of the mucous membrane
    b. Fluid level
    c. Thickening of the sinus lining
    d. Thickening of the sinus lining and fluid level

95. Empyema refers to:
    a. Swelling of mucous glands
    b. A tumour involving sebaceous glands
    c. A cavity filled with pus
    d. A connective tissue tumour

96. Antral polyps occur due to:
    a. Foreign bodies
    b. Displaced roots
    c. Hypertrophy of the mucosal lining
    d. Calcification of the mucous glands

97. Among the following, which may not be a tumour involving the maxillary sinus?
    a. Squamous cell carcinoma
    b. Basal cell carcinoma
    c. Adenoid cystic carcinoma
    d. Adenocarcinoma

98. Masseter is palpated at:
    a. Maxillary tuberosity region
    b. Lateral aspect of the ramus of the mandible
    c. Medial aspect of the body of the mandible
    d. Chin region

99. Medial pterygoid muscle is palpated at:
    a. Medial aspect of the mandible
    b. Medial aspect of the maxilla
    c. Lateral aspect of the mandible
    d. Lateral aspect of the maxilla

100. Lateral pterygoid muscle is palpated at:
    a. Medial aspect of the mandible
    b. Medial aspect of the maxilla
    c. Maxillary tuberosity region
    d. Over the temporal fascia

Ans. 94. a 95. c 96. c 97. b 98. b 99. a 100. c

SECTION XI

1. Displacement of the articular disk of the TMJ occurs in which direction?
   a. Anteromedially
   b. Anteroposteriorly
   c. Anterolaterally
   d. Anteriorly

2. Clicking of the TMJ indicates:
   a. Displaced condyle
   b. Rubbing of condyle with glenoid fossa
   c. Disk displacement with reduction
   d. Disk displacement without reduction

3. Reciprocal clicking of TMJ refers to:
   a. Bilateral clicking of the TMJ
   b. Unilateral clicking of the TMJ
   c. Clicking while opening the mouth
   d. Clicking while closing the mouth

4. Among the following statements about degenerative joint disease, which is incorrect?
   a. It is an inflammatory TMJ disorder
   b. Chronic microtrauma may be a cause
   c. Parafunctional habits can be a contributory factor
   d. It is usually unilateral

5. One of the features of Still's disease is:
   a. Stomatitis
   b. Ulcerations of the mouth
   c. Micrognathia
   d. Macroglossia

6. Usually in case of condylar fractures, the condyle gets displaced:
   a. Laterally and posteriorly
   b. Medially and anteriorly
   c. Laterally and anteriorly
   d. Medially and posteriorly

Ans. 1. a 2. c 3. d 4. a 5. c 6. b

7. Formation of granulation tissue in the TMJ is seen in:
   a. Degenerative joint disease
   b. Rheumatoid arthritis
   c. MPDS
   d. Condylar hyperplasia

8. "Phossy jaw" is associated with:
   a. Hyperparathyroidism
   b. Phosphorus poisoning
   c. Metastatic jaw involvement
   d. Multiple myeloma

9. Black hairy tongue is due to hypertrophy of:
   a. Filiform papillae
   b. Fungiform papillae
   c. Circumvallate papillae
   d. Foliate papillae

10. Auric stomatitis is due to:
    a. Gold poisoning
    b. Silver poisoning
    c. Mercury poisoning
    d. Arsenic poisoning

11. Pink's disease is also called as:
    a. Micrognathia
    b. Ectodermal dysplasia
    c. Discoid lupus erythematosus
    d. Acrodynia

12. Acrodynia refers to:
    a. Gold poisoning
    b. Arsenic poisoning
    c. Silver poisoning
    d. Mercury poisoning

13. Plumbism refers to:
    a. Gold poisoning
    b. Lead poisoning
    c. Mercury poisoning
    d. Silver poisoning

Ans. 7. b 8. b 9. a 10. a 11. d 12. d 13. b

14. The disease characterized by café-au-lait spots and sessile or pedunculated tumours of the skin and mucous membrane is:
    a. Peutz-Jeghers syndrome
    b. Von Recklinghausen's disease
    c. Albright's syndrome
    d. Pink's disease
15. Among the following, which is not a feature of Albright's syndrome?
    a. Café-au-lait spots
    b. Precocious puberty
    c. Polyostotic fibrous dysplasia
    d. Fissured tongue
16. Chloasma refers to:
    a. Excessive accumulation of cholesterol
    b. Pigmentation associated with pregnancy
    c. Connective tissue tumour
    d. Tumour affecting the adipose tissue
17. Pregnancy-associated pigmentation is seen in:
    a. First trimester b. Second trimester
    c. Third trimester d. After pregnancy.
18. Which is the disease associated with pigmentation of the oral mucosa and polyposis of the small intestine?
    a. Peutz-Jeghers syndrome
    b. Albright's syndrome
    c. Von Recklinghausen's disease
    d. Still's discase
19. Increase in flow of thick saliva, metallic taste, itching of the mouth and cracking or swelling of the lips are features of:
    a. Argyria
    b. "Phossy jaw"
    c. Mercurialism
    d. Quinine drug therapy
20. Adrenal insufficiency results in:
    a. Cushing's syndrme
    b. Addison's disease
    c. Albright's syndrome
    d. Diabetes insipidus

Ans. 14. b 15. d 16. b 17. c 18. a 19. c 20. b

21. Among the following, which is not a feature of Cushing's syndrome?
    a. Adiposis of the upper part of the body
    b. Buffalo hump
    c. Pigmentation in the oral cavity
    d. Vascular hypertension

22. Aldosterone promotes:
    a. Sodium retention
    b. Sodium excretion
    c. Potassium retention
    d. Calcium retention

23. Glycosuria and albuminuria are features of:
    a. Cushing's syndrome
    b. Albright's syndrome
    c. Addison's disease
    d. Diabetes mellitus

24. Burning sensation of the mouth can be a feature in:
    a. Pregnancy
    b. Menstruation
    c. Diabetes mellitus
    d. Hypertension

25. Among the following, which is not an action of insulin?
    a. Promotion of glucose uptake in the liver
    b. Promotion of production and release of glucose
    c. Synthesis of fatty acids in the adipose tissue
    d. Decreasing plasma glucose level

Ans. 21. c 22. a 23. a 24. c 25. b